AF811444

Morgenroth · Kozuschek, Pancreatitis

With compliments

SOLVAY

SOLVAY PHARMACEUTICAL GROUP

Konrad Morgenroth · Waldemar Kozuschek

Pancreatitis

In cooperation with Jürgen Hotz

Illustrated by Gerhard Pucher

Walter de Gruyter
Berlin · New York 1991

Prof. Dr. med. Konrad Morgenroth
Ruhr-Universität Bochum
Institut für Pathologie
Universitätsstraße 150
D-4630 Bochum-Querenburg

Prof. Dr. med. Waldemar Kozuschek
Chirurgische Klinik
Knappschaftskrankenhaus
Bochum-Langendreer-Universitätsklinik
In der Schornau
D-4630 Bochum

Prof. Dr. med. Jürgen Hotz
Allgemeines Krankenhaus Celle
Siemens-Platz 4
D-3100 Celle

© Copyright 1991 by Walter de Gruyter & Co., Berlin 30. All rights reserved, including those of translation into foreign languages. No part of this book may be reproduced in any form – by photoprint, microfilm or any other means nor transmitted nor translated into a machine language without written permission from the publisher.

Medical science is constantly developing. Research and clinical experience expand our knowledge, especially with regard to treatment and medication.

For dosages and applications mentioned in this work, the reader may rely on the authors, editors and publisher having taken great pains to ensure that these indications reflect the standard of knowledge at the time this work was completed.

Nevertheless, all users are requested to check the package leaflet of the medication, in order to determine for themselves whether the recommendations given for the dosages or the likely contraindications differ from those given in this book. This is especially true for medication which is seldom used or has recently been put on the market and for medication whose application has been restricted by the German Ministry of Health.

The quotation of registered names, trade names, trade marks, etc. in this copy does not imply, even in the absence of specific statement that such names are exempt from laws and regulations protecting trade marks, etc. and therefore free for gerneral use.

Cover design: Rudolf Hübler, Berlin
Typesetting and Printing: Appl, Wemding.
Binding: Lüderitz & Bauer GmbH, Berlin.
Printed in Germany.

Preface

The number of cases of acute or chronic pancreatitis is constantly rising. On the other hand technical advances during the past few years have increased the possiblities in diagnosis and treatment of pancreatitis. This group of diseases is a challenge requiring an interdisciplinary approach concerning almost every medical field.

In the present book a clinico-pathomorphological synopsis is being attempted. A visual impression of the formal pathogenetic course of the disease in relation to the clinical symptoms is to be imparted by the presentation of light- and electron microscopically tangible alterations. They constitute the results of close cooperation between gastroenterologists, radiologists, surgeons and pathologists.

The rendition of the light- and electron microscopical findings are supplemented by a number of three-dimensional reproductions, which take the functional parameters into consideration in most points. They were made by the graphic artist Gerhard Pucher, who produced them combining superb technique with a great deal of sensitivity for the problem. We are particularly grateful to him for his contributions, especially to this book, and his cooperation, which has proven to be invaluable for many years.

We also thank our former doctorands Dr. M. Luka, Dr. W. Rambach and Dr. Rogenwallner, for the good teamwork. We are indebted to Dr. P. Schlichting (Radiology Department of the Knappschafts-Krankenhaus Bochum-Langendreer-University Clinic) for access to and selection of the radio- and computerized tomographs.

Our special thanks goes to the Walter de Gruyter publishing company and their staff for their support in the realization and the excellent endowment of the book, in which all of our wishes were taken into consideration.

Bochum, 1991

K. Morgenroth
W. Kozuschek

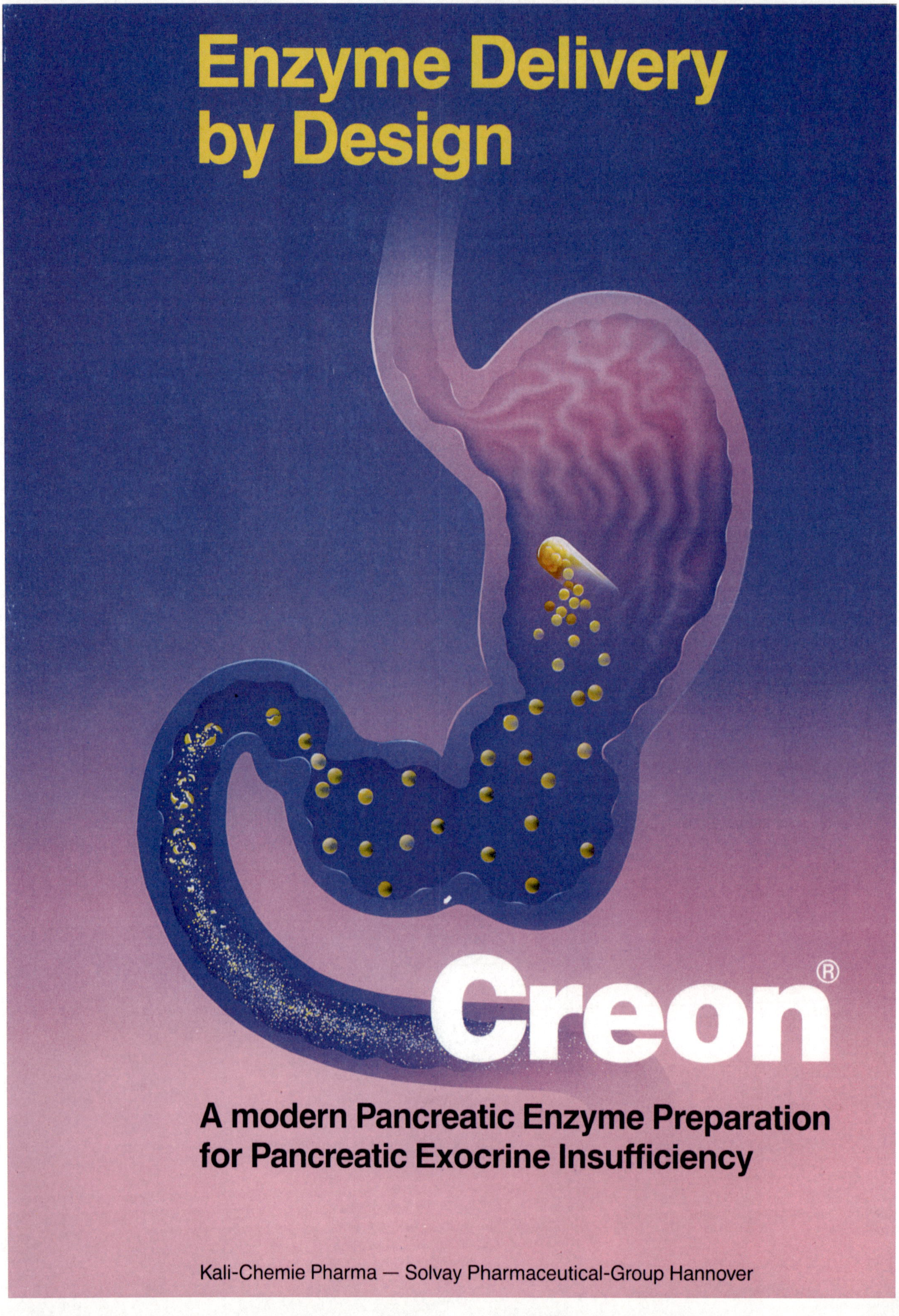
Enzyme Delivery
by Design
Creon®
A modern Pancreatic Enzyme Preparation
for Pancreatic Exocrine Insufficiency
Kali-Chemie Pharma — Solvay Pharmaceutical-Group Hannover

Contents

1 Introduction

Although in ancient Greece doctors were familiar with the pancreas, calling it παν κρεασ, all flesh (Schirmer 1893), the anatomical structure and physiology of the organ were first discovered relatively late. The efferent duct in man was described by Johann Georg Wirsung in 1642. Following almost complete removal of the pancreas in the dog by Johann Konrad Brunner (1688), it was general opinion for a long time that the pancreas was not a vital organ. Only through the experimental studies of Claude Bernard (1856), who first induced pancreatitis in a dog and discovered the effect of lipase, did interest for this organ flourish.

The acute necrosis of the pancreas with fat necrosis was first described by Balser (1882) and successfully surgically treated by von Körte (1894). Chiari (1883) believed that acute pancreatitis was due to intrapancreatic activation of the proteolytic enzymes and thus developed the theory of tryptic autodigestion of the organ, which has been confirmed by a large number of experimental and clinical investigations and has proven to be the essential pathogenetic principle until present day.

Observations during the last decades have shown that the number of cases of acute and chronic pancreatitis is increasing (Hoefler 1979). The introduction of diagnostic methods such as endoscopic retrograde cholangiopancreatography (ERCP), sonography and computerized tomography have opened new possibilities for investigation of this organ and its diseases. The understanding of the formal and causal pathogenesis of acute and chronic inflammation could be increased considerably by new discoveries in the micromorphology, morbid anatomy and clinical chemistry, by determination and verification of the interactions between structure and functions. On the basis of these findings effective conservative and surgical therapeutical concepts have been acquired.

Aside from the presentation of the clinical picture, diagnostics and the treatment of acute and chronic pancreatitis, comparison of morphological findings of the normal and disturbed structure of the pancreas obtained by different methods should provide a visual impression of the formal pathogenesis of inflammatory diseases of the pancreas.

2 Normal Structure and Function of the Exocrine Pancreas

(Figs. 1–17)

In man the pancreas develops from a larger dorsal and smaller ventral primordium, which fuse in the 12 mm embryo due to migration of the ventral primordium. These rudiments form a belt-like structure, the hepatopancreatic ring, from the intestinal epithelium of the duodenal area. The efferent duct in the dorsal primordium forms the main pancreatic duct or duct of Wirsung. From the duct of the ventral primordium the accessory duct or duct of Santorini develops, either sharing a duodenal orifice with the duct of Wirsung or having one of its own at the minor duodenal papilla (Langmann 1979, Ferner 1979).

The rarely occurring malformations of the pancreas, in the form of the annular pancreas or divisum, originate from the initially separate ventral or dorsal primordia. The frequently arising heterotopias of pancreatic tissue result from the general hereditary ability of the midintestine to produce pancreatic parenchyma (Ferner 1979, Remmele 1984).

In the adult the pancreas weighs 70 to 90 g and measures 13 to 15 cm in length. It is located in the retroperitoneum ventral to the second lumbar vertebra. It extends from the convexity of the duodenum to the hilus of the spleen. The head of the gland (Caput pancreatis) is distinguished from the body and tail (Cauda pancreatis). The approximately 12 cm long main pancreatic duct runs closer to the dorsal wall of the organ than the ventral surface. It receives tributaries and joins the common bile duct to form with it a common orifice upon the major duodenal papilla (Ferner 1979). From the evolution of the organ it becomes understandable that considerable variations in the orificial situation can exist in the ductal system. Three basic forms can be distinguished from one another. In 60 to 70% there is a Y-shaped orifice with a common final stretch between the pancreatic and choledochal ducts. In 20 to 30% there is a V-shaped orifice of the neighboring ducts and in 10 to 20% a U-shaped, separate orifice in the papilla. The terminal stretch of the common bile duct runs through a ridge in the head of the pancreas in 40% and in 15% it is completely surrounded by pancreatic tissue, so that in pancreatitis stenosis of the common bile duct can arise (Borchard 1987).

The arterial supply of the head of the pancreas occurs via a corona of anastomoses. The superior pancreatoduodenal arteries start from the common hepatic artery. The inferior pancreatoduodenal artery arises from the superior mesenterial artery. Body and tail of the gland are supplied by the pancreatic tributaries of the splenic artery. The veins running alongside of the arteries empty into the portal vein.

The pancreas is richly innervated. The nerves are arranged in perivascular, periacinar and perinsular networks (Radke et al. 1985). Empty synaptic vesicles or vesicles with dense contents are located at nerve endings and axons in the areas closest to the acinar cells. Enzyme histochemical and immunohistochemical findings allow the presumption that many of these nerves are of cholinergic nature (Schiebler 1987). Nerve fibres containing vasoactive peptide or gastrin-releasing polypeptide have also been demonstrated (Schiebler 1987) along with nerve fibres containing cholecystokinin-related peptide, neuropeptide or catecholamine.

The exocrine pancreas is presumably subject to nerval control (Schiebler 1987), because receptors for a large number of neurotransmitters are located at the basolateral cell membranes of the acinar cells.

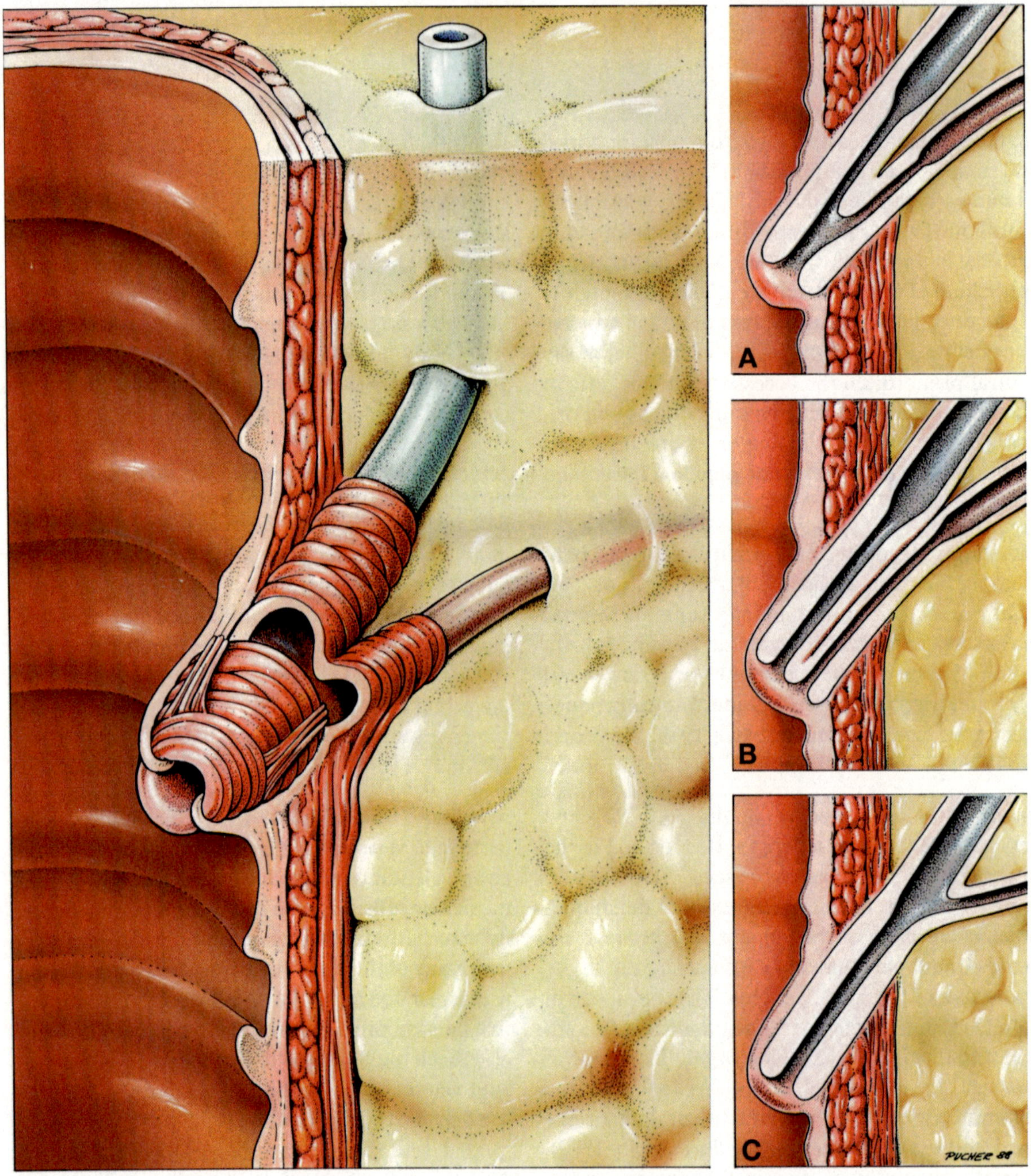

Fig. 1
Schematic presentation of the orifice of the ductal system of the pancreas, the common bile duct and its variations. 3 basic forms can be distinguished from one another.
A = V-shaped orifice of the neighboring ducts (20–30%)
B = U-shaped, separate orifices in the papilla (10–20%)
C = Y-shaped orifice with common final stretch between the pancreatic duct and the common bile duct (60–70%)

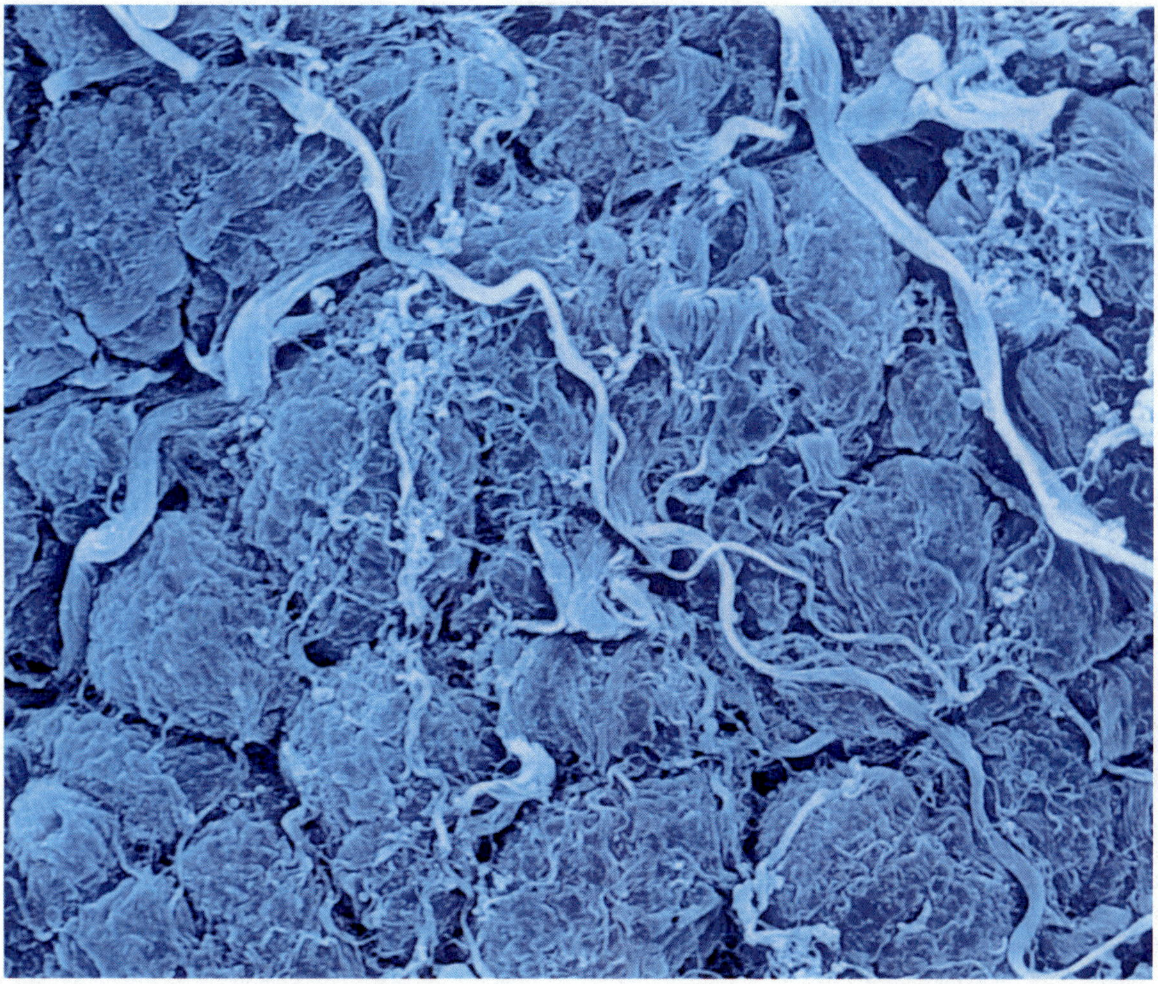

Fig. 2
Lobular and acinar structure of the pancreas. The individual acini are embedded in a loose connective tissue framework, in which blood vessels and nerves run
Scanning electron micrograph
Magnification: 800 ×

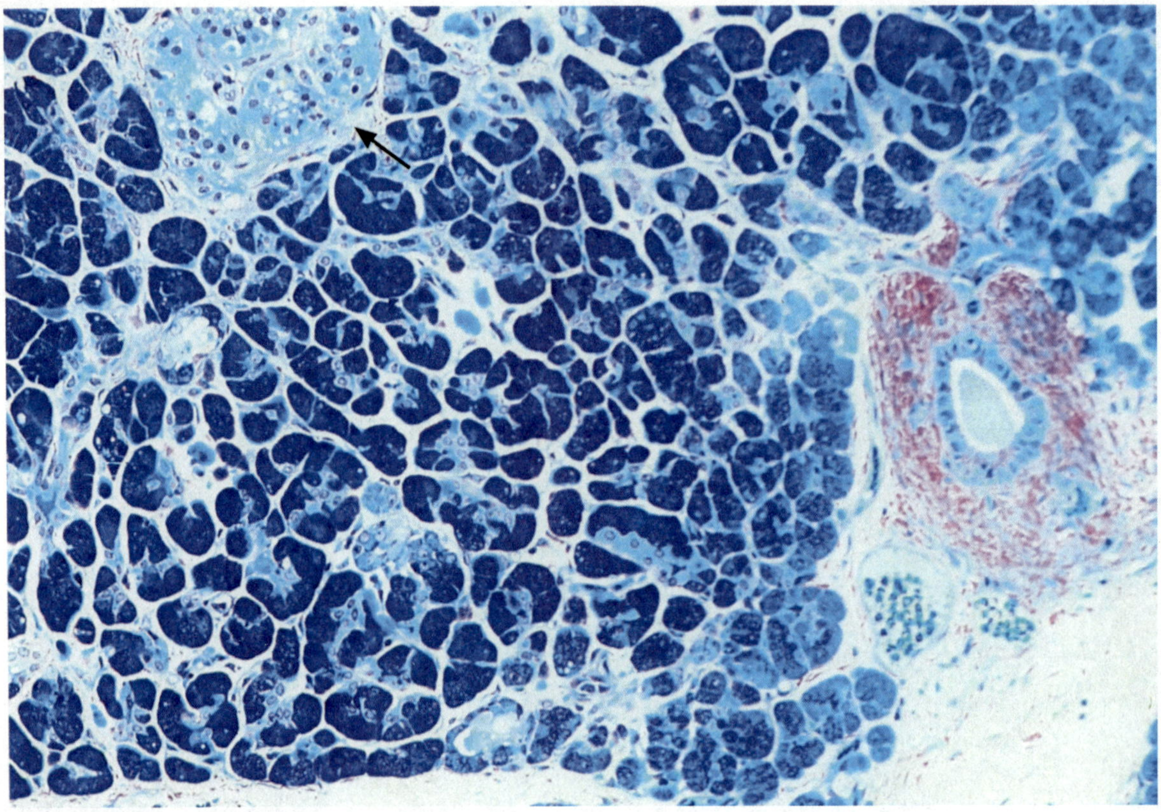

Fig. 3
Lobular and acinar structure of the pancreas. The lobuli are separated by a loose zone of connective tissue. Between the individual acini a loose fibrous structure, in which the capillaries supplying the acini run. At the upper edge of the picture (arrow) pancreatic islet. At the right edge of the picture cross section of efferent duct with periductal fibre zone.
Light micrograph
Semithin section
Stain: basic fuchsin and methylene blue
Magnification: 220 ×

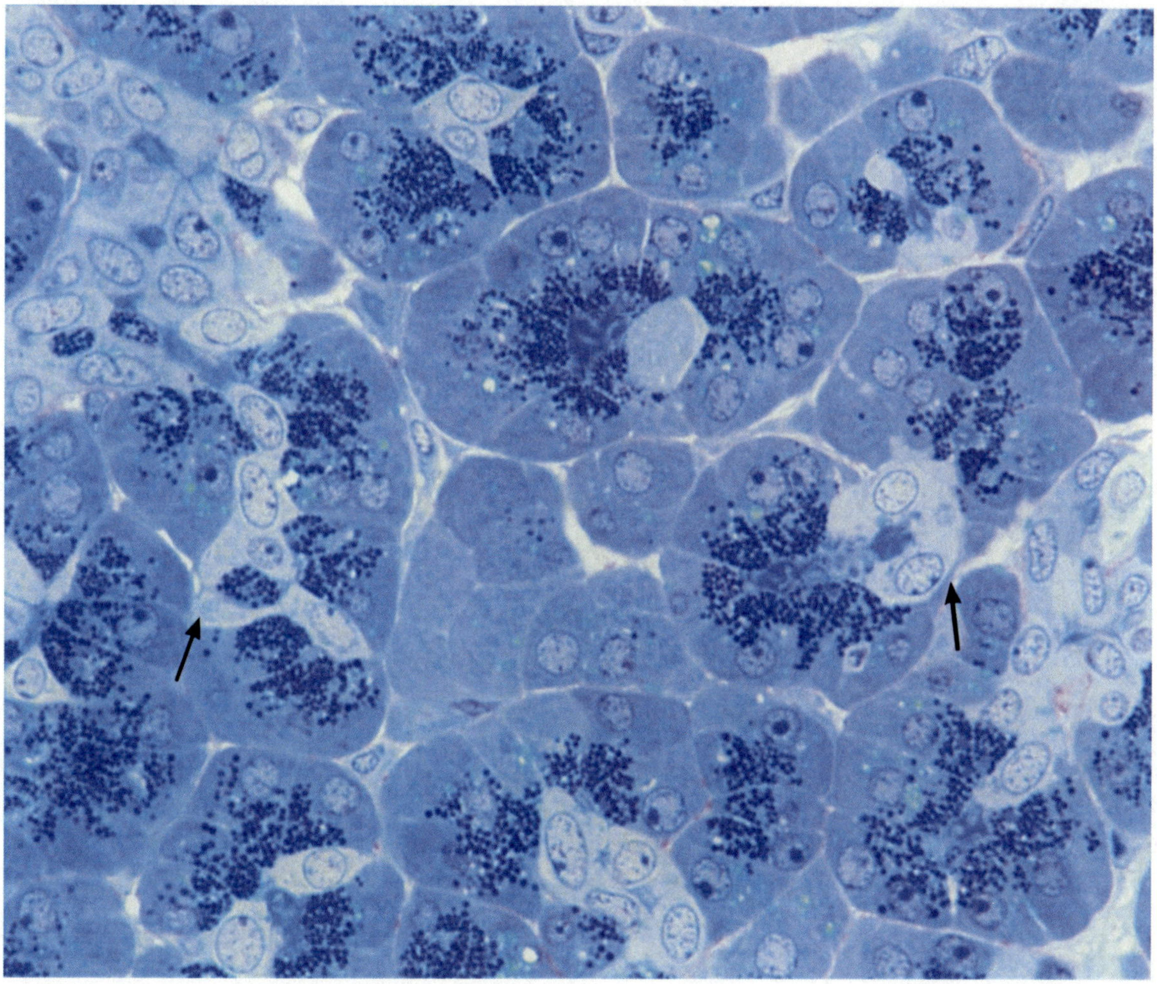

Fig. 4
Exocrine pancreas. The individual acini consist of pyramid-shaped epithelial cells with centrally aligned nuclei generally exhibiting conspicuous nucleoli. In the apical region of the epithelial cell densely packed zymogen granula. In the central parts of the individual acini centro-acinar cells with pale cytoplasm and oval, loosely arranged nuclei (arrows)
Light micrograph
Semithin section
Stain: basic fuchsin and methylene blue
Magnification: 740 ×

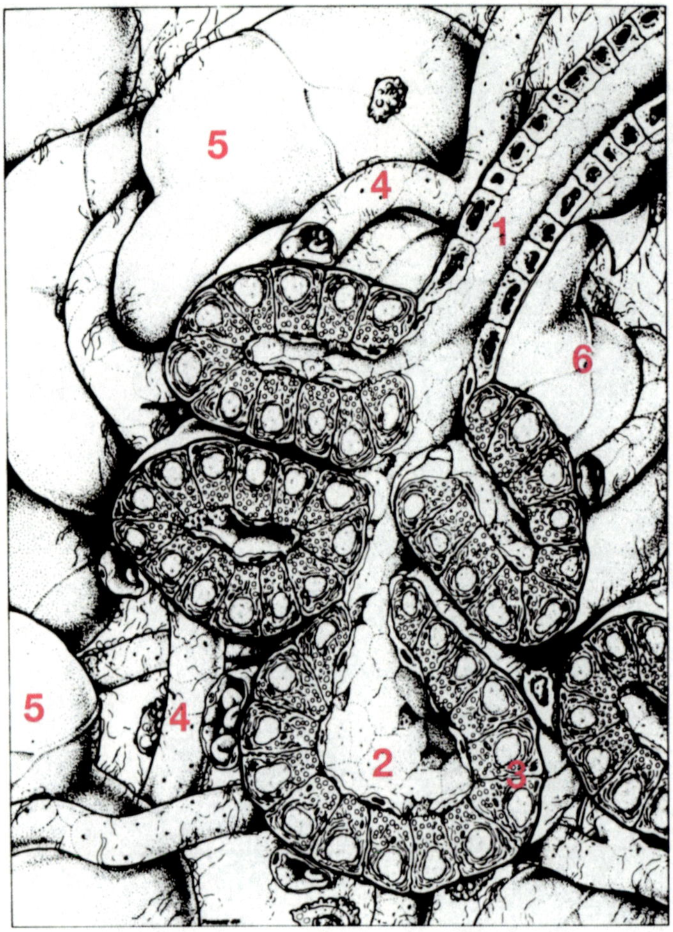

Fig. 5
Three-dimensional reproduction of the acinar system of the exocrine pancreas. The acinar lumina are lined by centro-acinar cells. Adjacent to the acinar lumina terminal branches of the duct system. Between the acini loosely arranged connective tissue framework with capillary network and nerve endings.
1 = efferent duct
2 = centro-acinar cells in an acinar lumen
3 = pyramidal acinar epithelial cells containing zymogen granula
4 = capillary network
5 = adjacent acini
6 = nerve endings

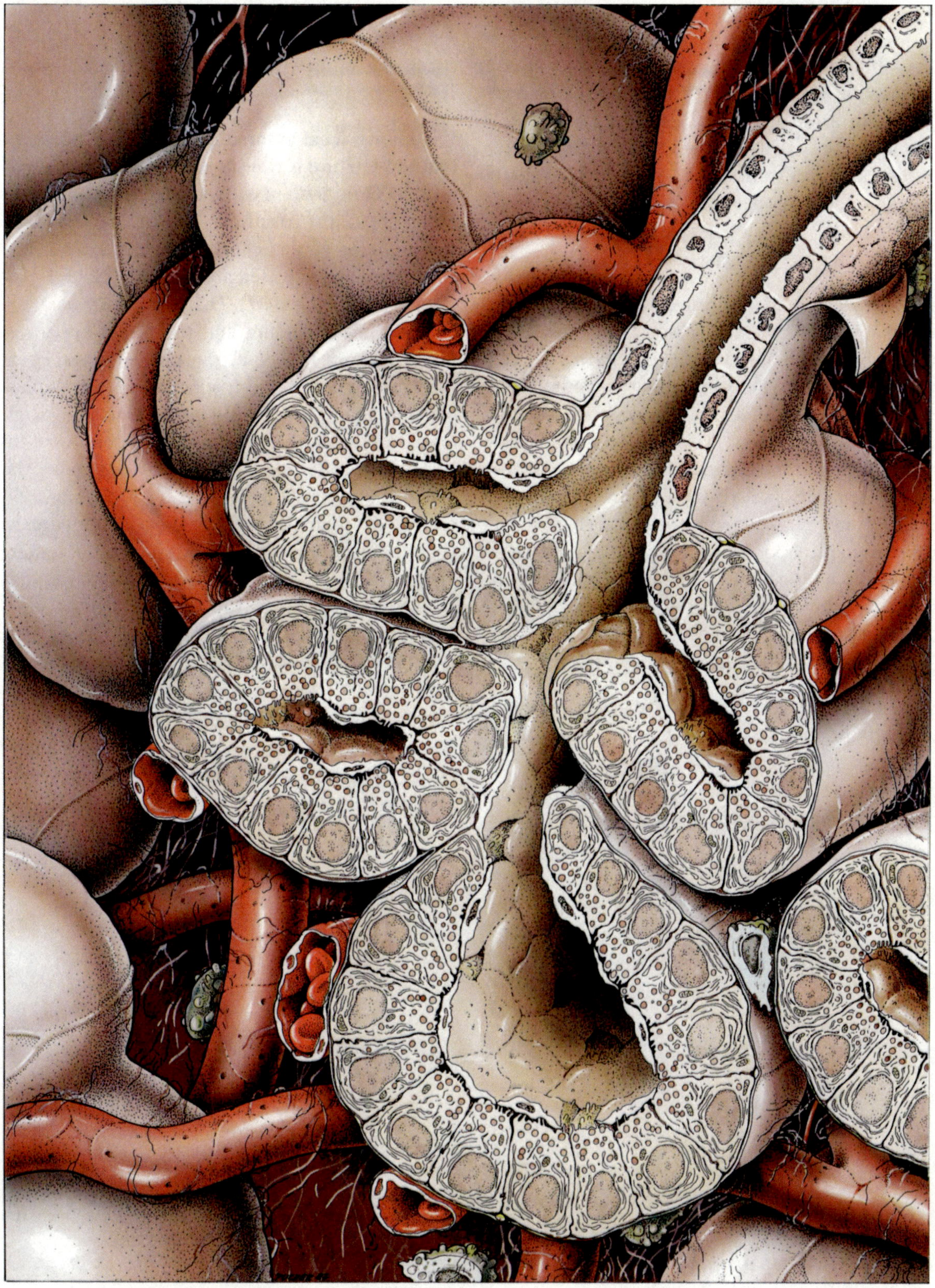

2.1 Acini (Figs. 2–11)

The lobuli of the exocrine pancreas consist of not always spherical and not only at the end of the ductal system arranged acini (Schiebler 1987). They form grape-like structures at the end of the ductal system. Connective tissue, in which blood vessels and nerves run, lies between the acini and the individual lobuli. Occasionally mast cells are interspersed in the perivascular fibrous tissue.

The acini are made of prismatic epithelial cells which border to a narrow lumen. There are a few narrow microvilli at the surface. Between the cell membranes of neighboring acinar cells there are contact zones exhibiting filamentary condensation of adjacent cytoplasm. A few individual desmosomes lie below. Round nuclei of constant size are located centrally in the cytoplasm of the epithelial cells. Round, homogeneously dense secretion granula lie in apical portions. The cytoplasm is rich in endoplasmic reticulum, which in part encloses the secretion droplets. In the cytoplasm mitochondria of the cristae type can be demonstrated. Larger Golgi fields lie in the perinuclear cytoplasm.

Synthesis of the secretions take place in the ribosomes of the endoplasmic reticulum (Palade 1975), which is a major constituent of the cytoplasm. The cisternal space of the endoplasmic reticulum is continuous space which is filled with a mixture consisting of newly synthesized proteins (Kern 1987).

It is known from autoradiographic investigations, that the mixture is transported to and transferred into the Golgi system within 15 to 20 minutes. The Golgi apparatus constitutes the second organelle system of the epithelial cells, in which synthesized substances are collected and undergo further processing (Rothman 1987). The passage between the endoplasmic reticulum and the Golgi apparatus takes place in so-called transport vesicles which bud from the ribosome-free parts of the endoplasmic reticulum following contact with the membranes of the Golgi apparatus with subsequent fusion with the latter. In the Golgi apparatus the proteins are sorted into different groups and directed to their functional purpose (Farquhar 1985). The proteins are enveloped by a coating membrane. The secretion granula probably undergo further maturation, the individual steps, however, are yet obscure (Mellmann et al. 1986). The zymogen granula migrate to the apical cell membrane which represent the border to the acinar lumen. The membranes of the zymogen granula fuse with the cell membrane, subsequently opening to the lumen allowing exocytosis of the contents into the lumen.

Fig. 6
Structure of the acinar system of the pancreas. Pyramidal acinar epithelial cells with densely packed zymogen granula in the apical regions. Rough endoplasmic reticulum densely packed in the cytoplasm. Adjacent individual mitochondria. Terminal branches of an efferent duct with transition to the centro-acinar area (arrow) of the section.
Transmission electron micrograph
Magnification: 5600 ×

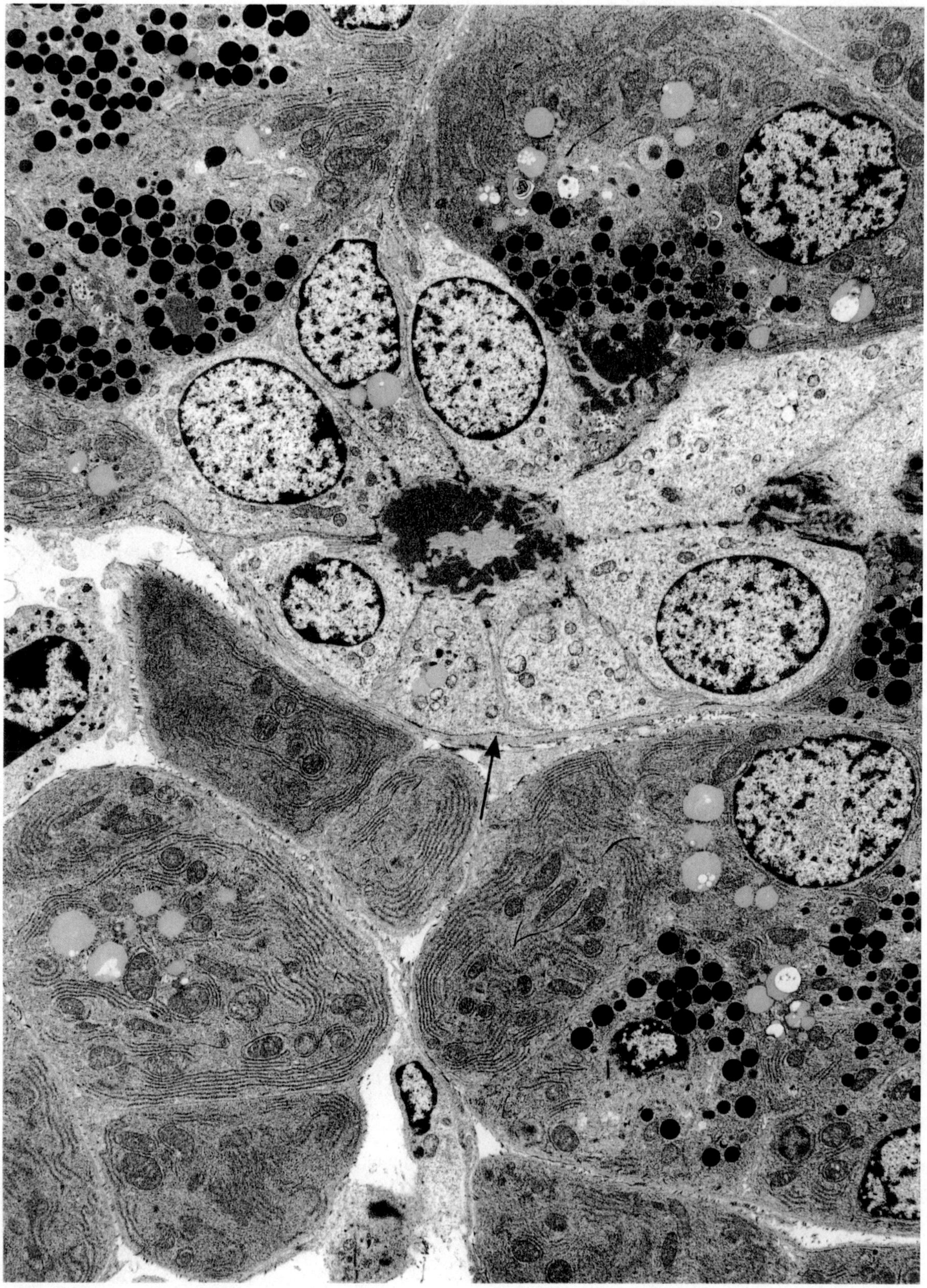

2.2 Epithelium of the Ductal System

The ducts of the pancreas are lined by columnar epithelial cells. The epithelial cells including the centro-acinar cells belonging to the ductal system all have a pale cytoplasm relatively lacking organelles. At the surface of the cells a relatively evenly distributed microvilli system can be demonstrated, which may perform receptor functions. In the apical regions of the cells between the cell membranes of the neighboring cells zonulae occludentes (tight junctions), further below zonulae adherentes and again below desmosomes exist. The cell membranes exhibit narrow cytoplasmic protrusions and basal indentations into the intercellular spaces.

Via the membraneous system of the duct epithelium transport of ions and water takes place, especially in the intralobular areas (Schiebler 1987). The ductal epithelium probably has special significance in bicarbonate secretion.

In all areas of the ductal system mucous secretion can be demonstrated. Even in intralobular ducts a few individual cubic mucous-secreting cells are interspersed in the epithelium. Mucous secretion takes place particularly in the larger interlobular regions and in the main efferent ducts. In the secretion-producing cells prosecretion granula are located especially in the apical cytoplasm. The mucous covers the surface. It is assumed (Schiebler 1987) that the mucous plays an important role in protecting the ductal epithelium from the influence of the pancreatic juices produced in the acini.

Until today the regulatory mechanisms of the function of the ductal epithelium remain obscure. The function is probably dependent on receptors and controlled by substances belonging to the secretin group and e.g. by acetylcholine, cholecystokinase and serotonin.

Fig. 7
Interstitium of the acinar system of the pancreas. Branches of nerve endings are arranged in a loose connective tissue framework (arrow). Adjacent a mast cell with typical, partially granular, partially lamellar contents.
Transmission electron micrograph
Magnification: 21 000 ×

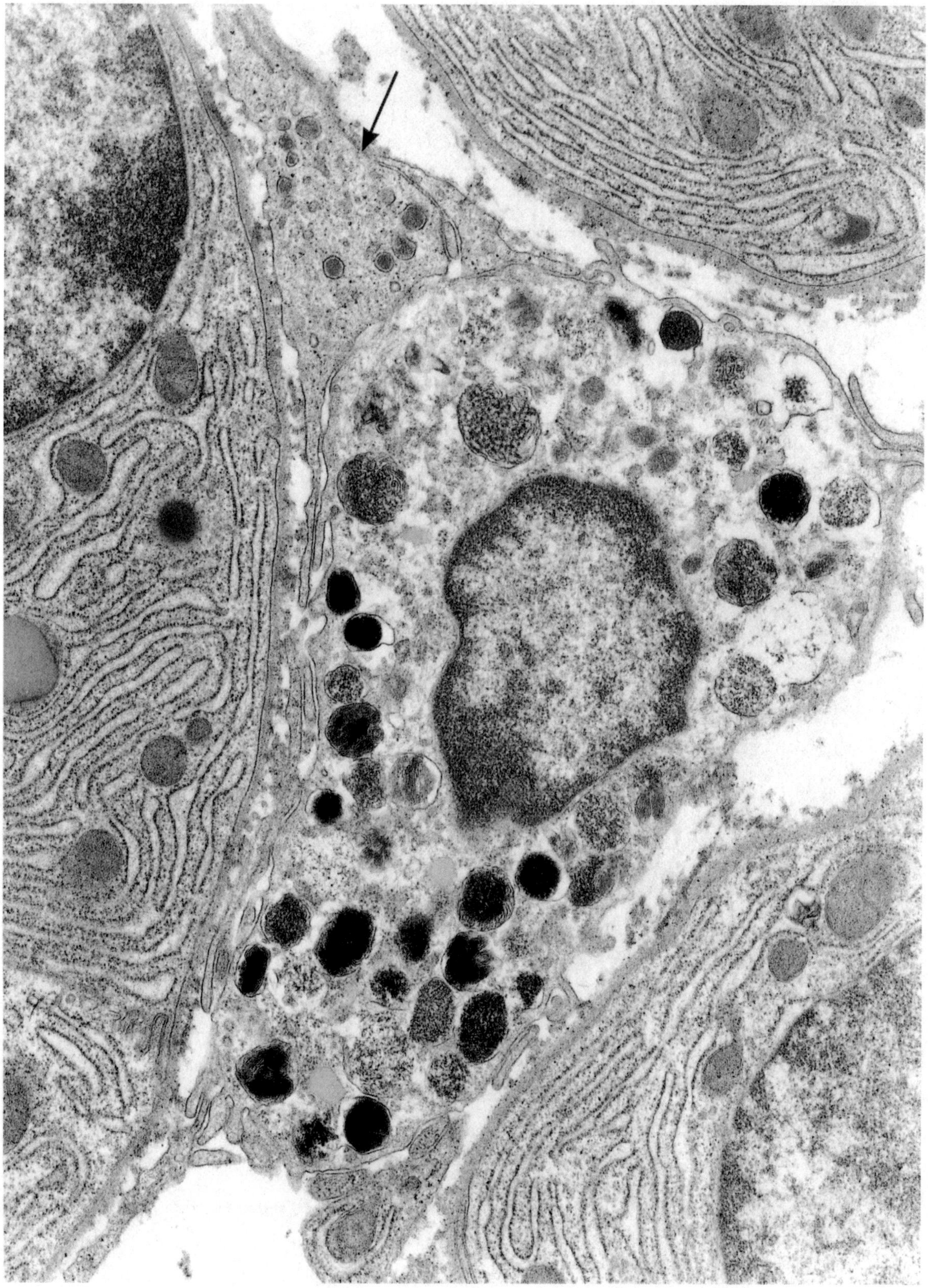

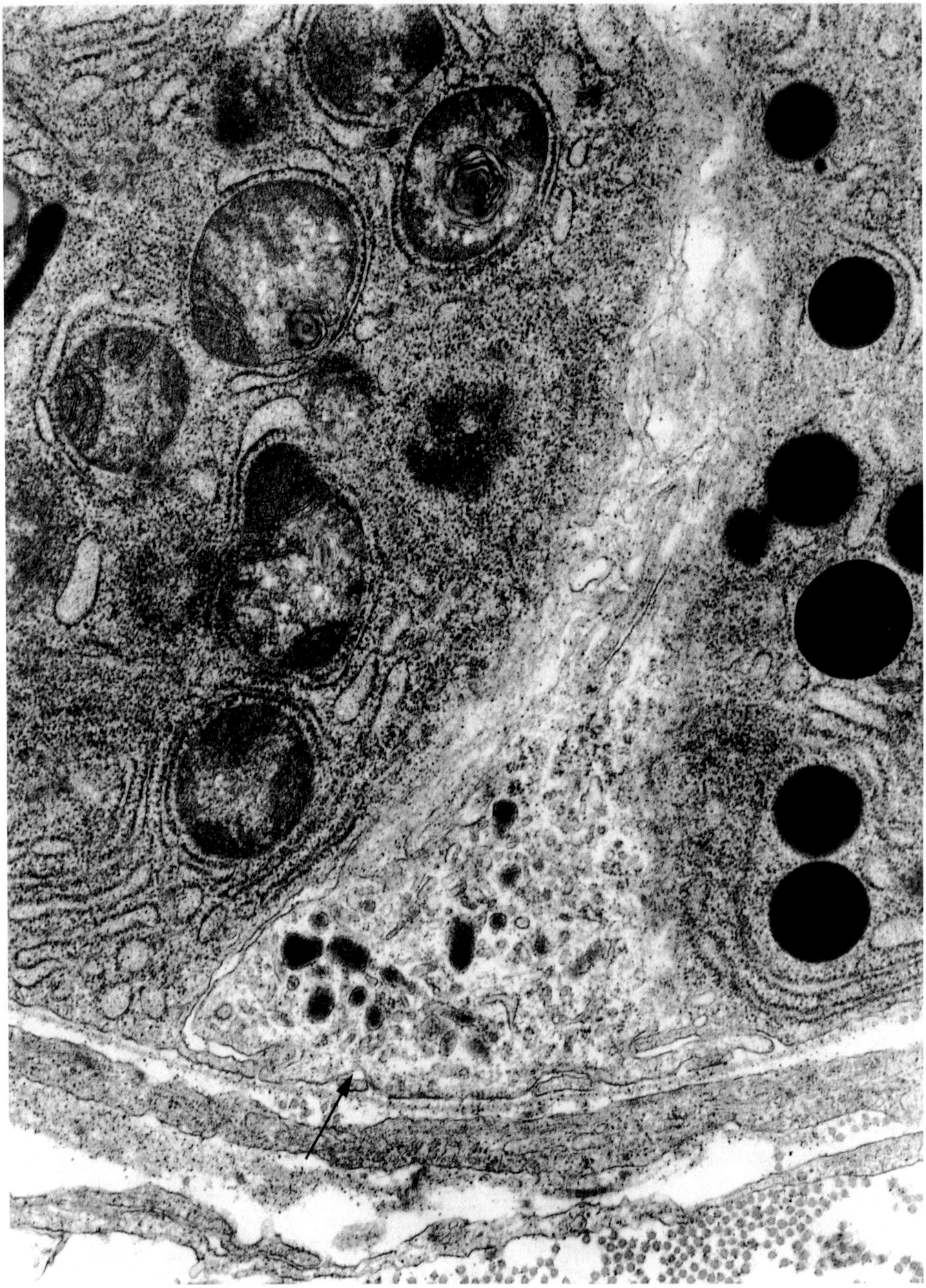

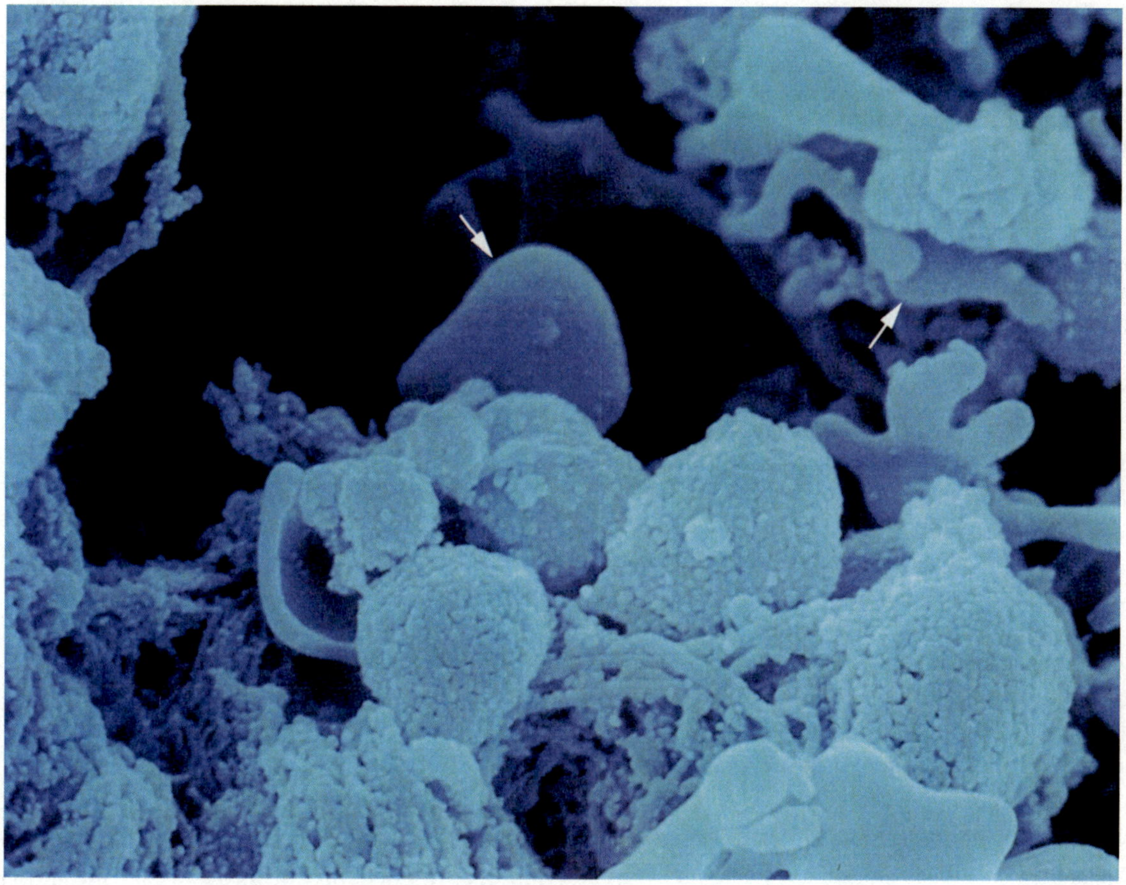

◁ Fig. 8
Nerval supply of the acinar system of the pancreas. Terminal nerve end branches penetrate the basement membrane and enter the acinar epithelium. The nerve endings lie immediately adjacent to the latero-basal parts of the cell membrane. In the section of the nerve endings typically differentiated neurosecretory granula (arrow).
Transmission electron micrograph
Magnification: 31 000 ×

Fig. 9
Intracytoplasmic structure of acinar cells. View into a partially opened acinar cell. In apical areas of the cell zymogen granula completely enveloped by rough endoplasmic reticulum. Inbetween a few individual lamella of endoplasmic reticulum and mitochondria of various sizes (arrow).
Scanning electron micrograph
Magnification: 33 000 ×

2.3 Physiology and Biochemistry of the Exocrine Pancreas

Approximately 1.5 to 2 l of pancreatic juices with a pH ranging between 8 and 8.5 is produced in the pancreas per day. Combined with the bile and the duodenal secretions the acidic chymus of the stomach is neutralized or shifted to a slightly alkaline pH (Schmidt and Thews 1980). In this neutral environment of the intestine the gastric pepsins are inactivated. The pancreatic secretions contain enzymes for fat-, carbohydrate- and protein digestion, the cations sodium, calcium, potassium and magnesium and the anions chloride, sulphate and phosphate. The enzymes for protein digestion are present as proenzymes trypsinogen, chymotrypsinogen, procarboxylpeptidase A and B as well as elastase. Trypsinogen is activated by the duodenal enterokinase by cleavage of a hexapeptide from the C-terminal. Activation of trypsin and the other proenzymes involved in protein digestion takes place autocatalytically by trypsin. Trypsin and chymotrypsin are endopeptidases. Of the enzymes available for fat digestion pancreatic lipase cleaves tri-. di- and monoglycerides into glycerine and fatty acids. The extremely stable pancreatic alpha-amylase for carbohydrate digestion does not need activation and cleaves alpha-glycoside compounds (Schmidt and Thews 1980, Remmele 1984).

Regulation of pancreatic secretion occurs in 3 phases:

1. The cephalic phase subsequent to viewing food as a reflex vagus stimulus
2. The gastric phase upon food ingestion into the stomach
3. The intestinal phase upon passage of gastric and fatty acids into the duodenum (Remmele 1984).

In the intestinal phase gastrointestinal hormones are released, which are produced in the S- and I-cells of the duodenum. In conjunction with calcium ions and AMP secretin causes excretion of large amounts of secretions with high bicarbonate and low enzyme content. Secretin is liberated in the duodenum upon entrance of gastric acid and reaches the cells of the excretory pancreas via the haemovascular system.

Liberation of the cholecystokinin-pancreozymin and gastrin is evoked by contact of peptones, amino acids and fats with the duodenal mucosa. Cholecystokinin-pancreozymin and gastrin cause secretion of a pancreas juice with high enzyme content (proteochylus). It also causes contraction and emptying of the gallbladder. Vasoactive peptide stimulates the exocrine glandular cells in a

Fig. 10
Cytoplasmic structure of the acinar cells. Narrow microvilli at the surface. The epithelial cells are only separated from one another by narrow intercellular spaces. In the apical cell regions tight junctions between the cell membranes of adjacent epithelial cells. In the basal regions of the acinar cells densely packed lamellar rough endoplasmic reticulum. Concentration of the zymogen granula in apical areas of the cell. From the basal to apical cytoplasm of the cell maturation of the secretions can be recognized due to the variable density of the granular character of the basic structures.
Transmission electron micrograph
Magnification: 13000 ×

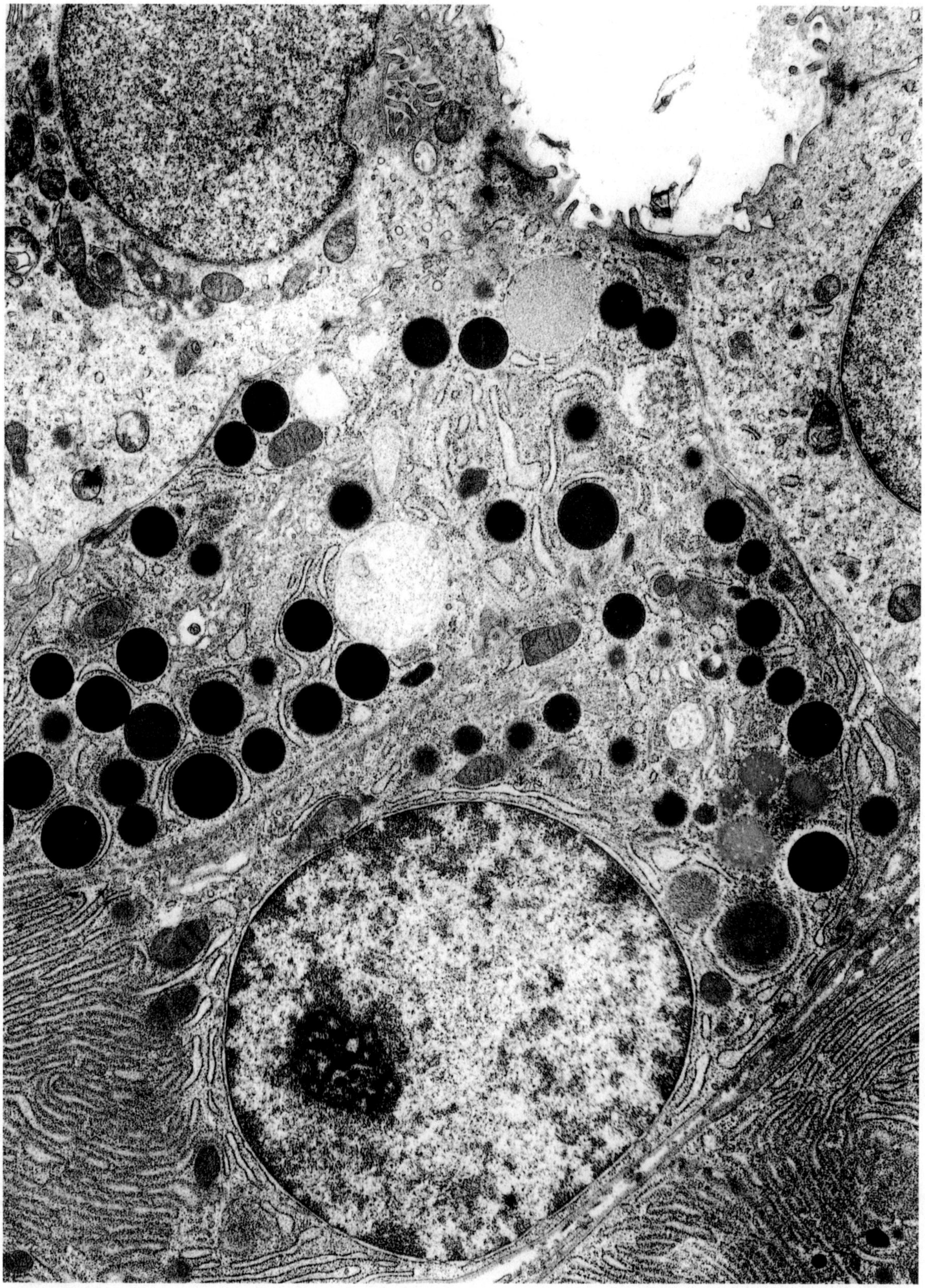

manner similar to secretin, but is weaker in strength. Somatostatin inhibits the secretion of bicarbonate and enzymes (Classen 1984).

Specific protease-inhibitors are produced in the pancreas to protect it from the enzymes produced by itself. In coalition with nonspecific trypsin-inhibitors present in the serum they prevent premature activation of the enzymes in the pancreatic parenchyma and the ductal system. Synthesis of the proteolytic enzymes as inactive zymogens and their storage in phospholipid membranes, the continual drainage of the secretions into the duodenum as well as the mucopolysaccharide layer covering the ductal epithelium are interpreted as further factors preventing autodigestion of the organ. Due to directed permeability of the acinar cell neither the enzymes nor their activators are capable of entering the cells during regular metabolism (Remmele 1984).

Fig. 11
Endoplasmic reticulum and mitochondria in the basal area of the cytoplasm of an acinar cell. Ribosomes are evenly distributed along the lamella of the endoplasmic reticulum. In the cytoplasm scattered droplets of neutral fat. Even structure of the cristae in the mitochondria.
Transmission electron micrograph
Magnification: 19000 ×

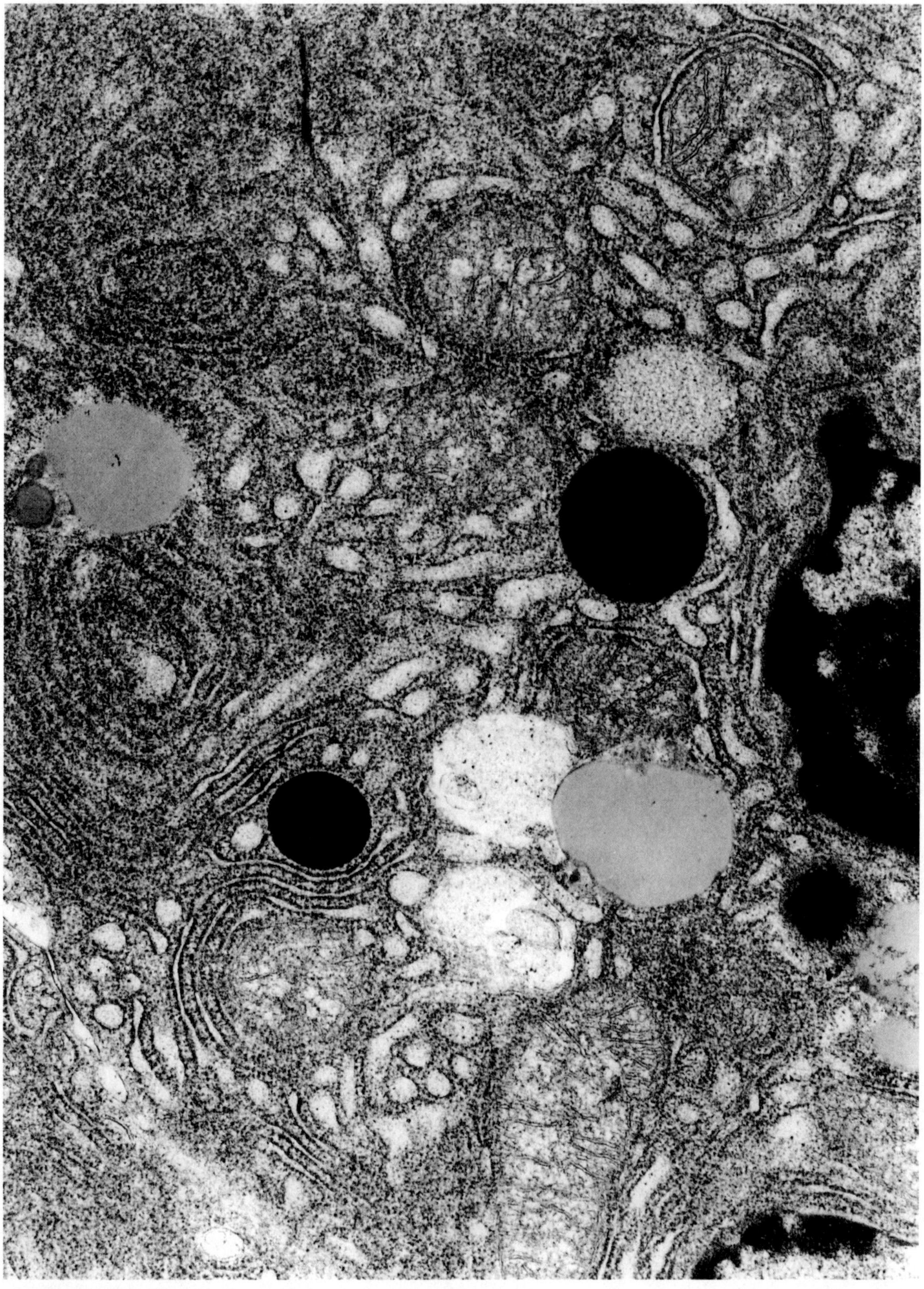

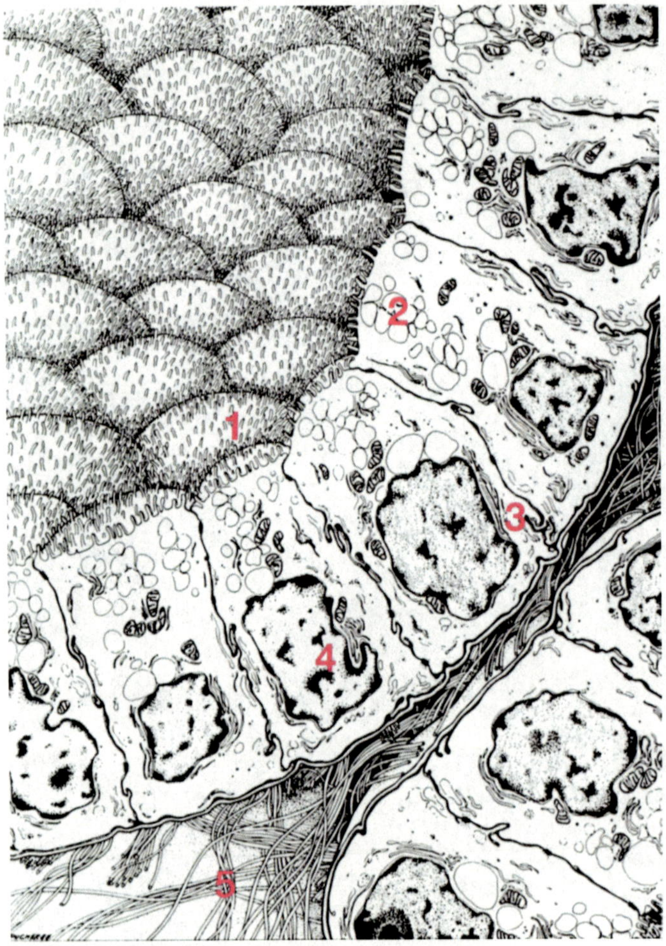

Fig. 12
Three-dimensional reproduction of the ductal epithelium. At the surface an even microvilli structure. Regular mosaic-like arrangement of the epithelial cells. Between the epithelial cells tight junctions in regular distribution in apical regions of the cell membranes. Below the epithelium a loose irregular network of fibres.

1 = Structure of microvilli
2 = Granula of prosecretions for mucous secretion in the epithelial cells
3 = Endoplasmic reticulum of the ductal epithelia
4 = Basal lamella of the ductal epithelium
5 = Subepithelial zone of connective tissue

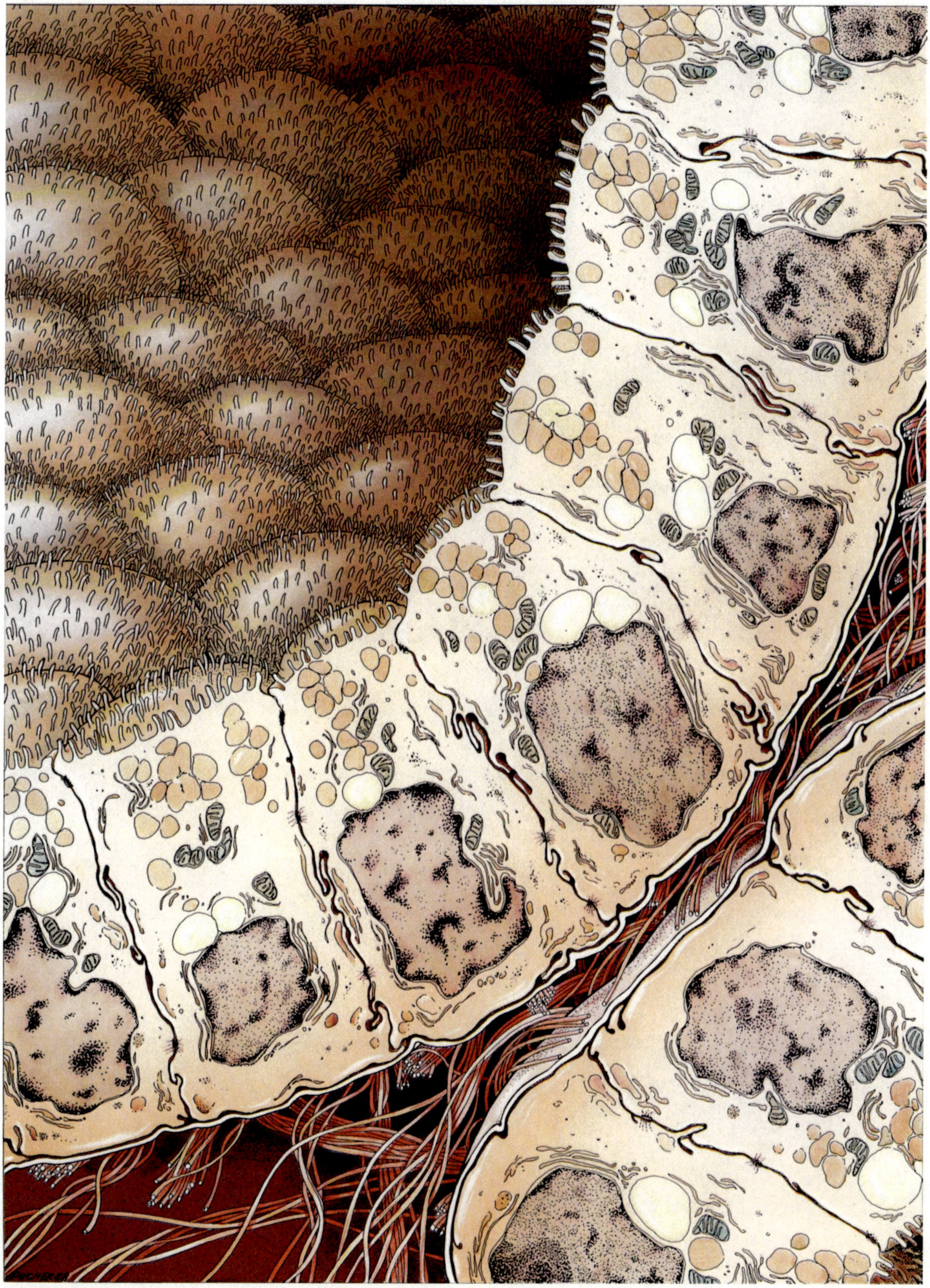

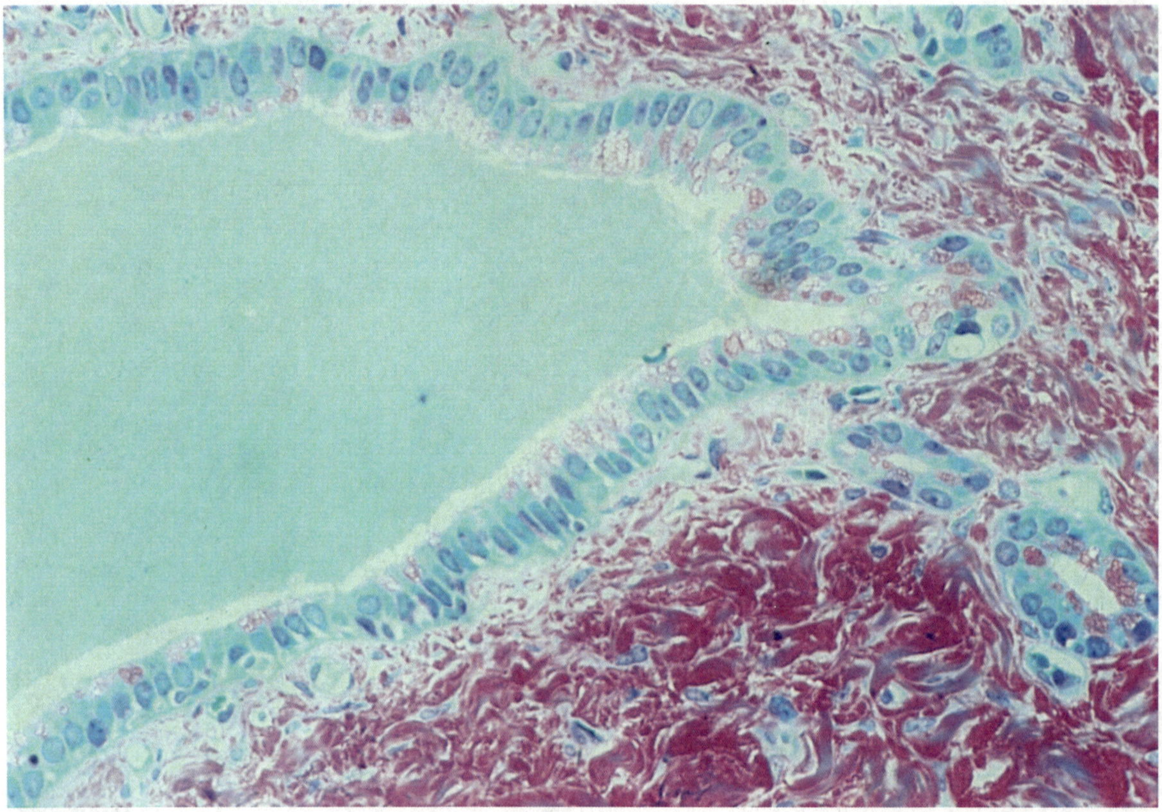

Fig. 13
Section of an efferent duct with regular lining by columnar epithelium. In the apical regions of the epithelium secretion complexes can be recognized. On the right side of the picture junction of a small ductal tributary. Regular periductal fibre zone.
Light micrograph
Semithin section
Stain: Basic fuchsin and methylene blue
Magnification: 660 ×

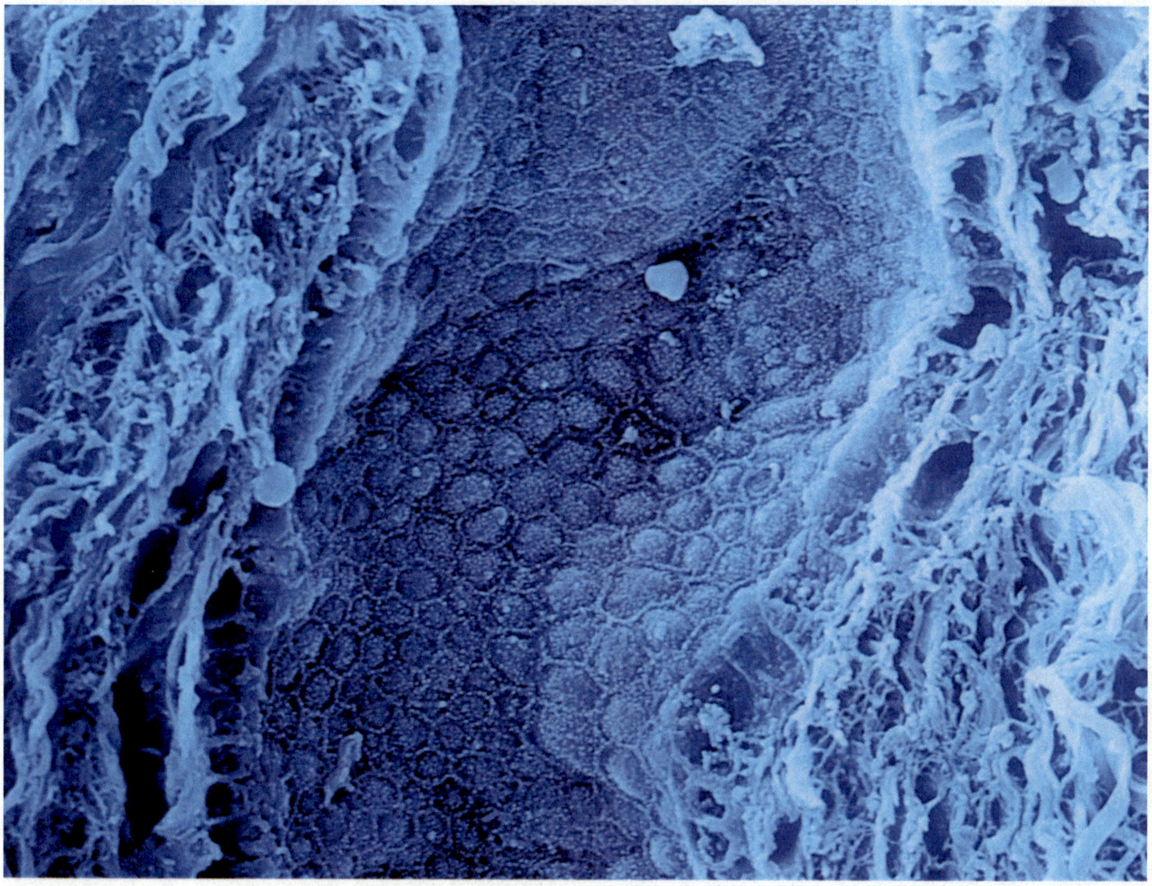

Fig. 14
Surface structure of the ductal epithelium in an efferent duct opened by tangential section. Regular mosaic-like surface structure of the epithelium. Slightly embossed border zones of the individual epithelial cells. Loose periductal fibre zone containing few blood vessels outside.
Scanning electron micrograph
Magnification: 11 000 ×

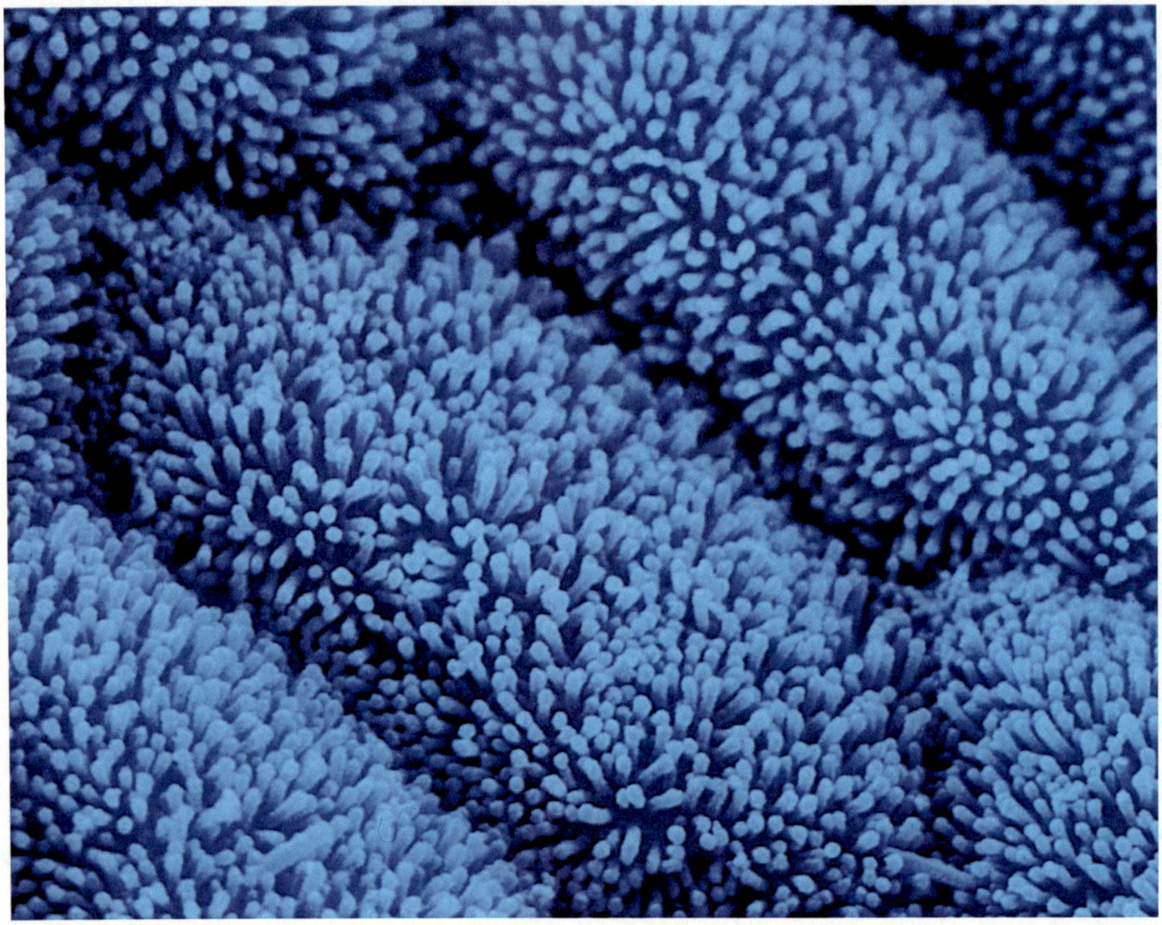

Fig. 15
Microvilli structure of the ductal epithelium. At the surface of the epithelial cells brush-like lining with cytoplasmic protrusions measuring 0.15 μm in diameter and each of equal length. Slight indentations of the surface membrane in vicinity of the cell borders.
Scanning electron micrograph
Magnification: 11000 ×

Fig. 16
Cytoplasmic structure of the epithelial cells of the ducts. In apical areas confluating granula of prosecretions of mucous (arrows). Between the epithelial cells narrow intercellular spaces with narrow cytoplasmic protrusions. Irregular condensation of the karyoplasm of the nuclei. ▷
Transmission electron micrograph
Magnification: 10000 ×

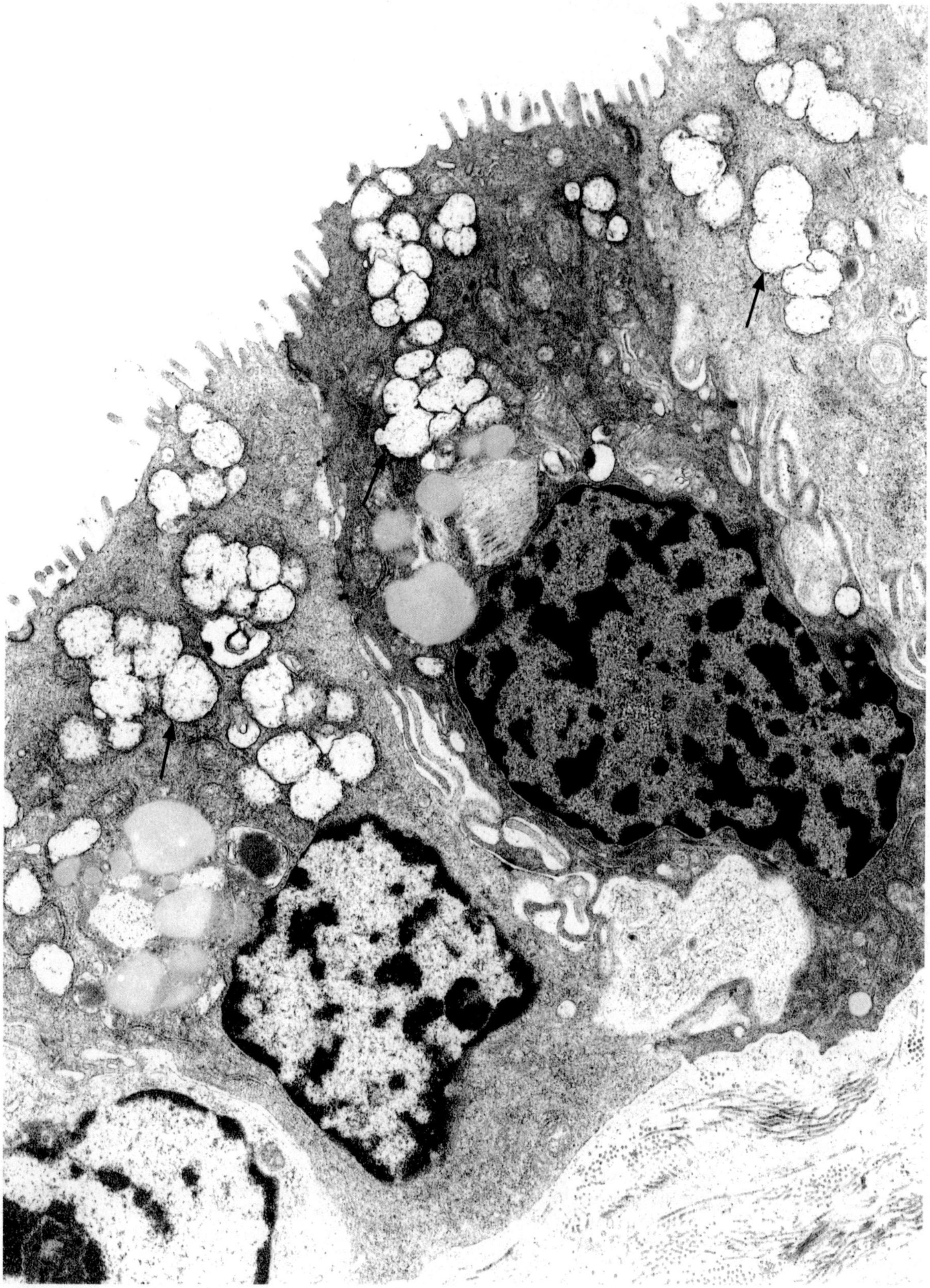

Table 1 Composition of pancreatic enzymes (Siegenthaler 1976)

Name	Effect and comments
Alpha-Amylase	cleaves polysaccharide to maltose, is secreted in its active form
Lipase	cleaves triglyceride to fatty acid and glycerine, is secreted in active form. Bile salts alter the pH-optimum into slightly acidic range and create optimal conditions for the effectivity of lipase
Sterolesterhydrolase	cleaves sterolesters, is secreted as an active enzyme, bile salts protect it from proteolytic inactivation
Phospholipase A	cleaves phosphatides at C2 into lysophosphatide and fatty acids, is secreted as a proenzyme
Phospholipase B	cleaves a further fatty acid from lysophosphatide at C1, is secreted as a proenzyme
Trypsin	an endopeptidase, which cleaves proteins and polypeptides within the molecule, prefers peptide bindings with Arg and Lys, is secreted in its inactivated form and is activated by enterokinase
Chymotrypsin A-C	are endopeptidases like trypsin, are activated by trypsin, can go through a series of already enzymatically active intermediate states during the process
Elastase	is an endopeptidase, digests elastin, is secreted as a proenzyme and is activated by trypsin
Collagenase	cleaves collagen
Kallikrein	liberates kallidin by proteolytic cleavage of kinogen, is secreted as kallikreinogen and is activated by trypsin
Carboxypeptidase A and B	cleave terminal amino acids from the C-terminal end of the peptide, activated by trypsin, Zn is coenzyme

Fig. 17
Cross section through fine branches of the ductal system. At the surface of the epithelial cells regular microvilli structure. The individual epithelial cells lie close to one another, separated only by narrow intercellular spaces. Regular nuclear structure. In the apical regions of the cytoplasm scattered prosecretion granula. Outside loose fibre structure.
Transmission electron micrograph
Magnification: 4600 ×

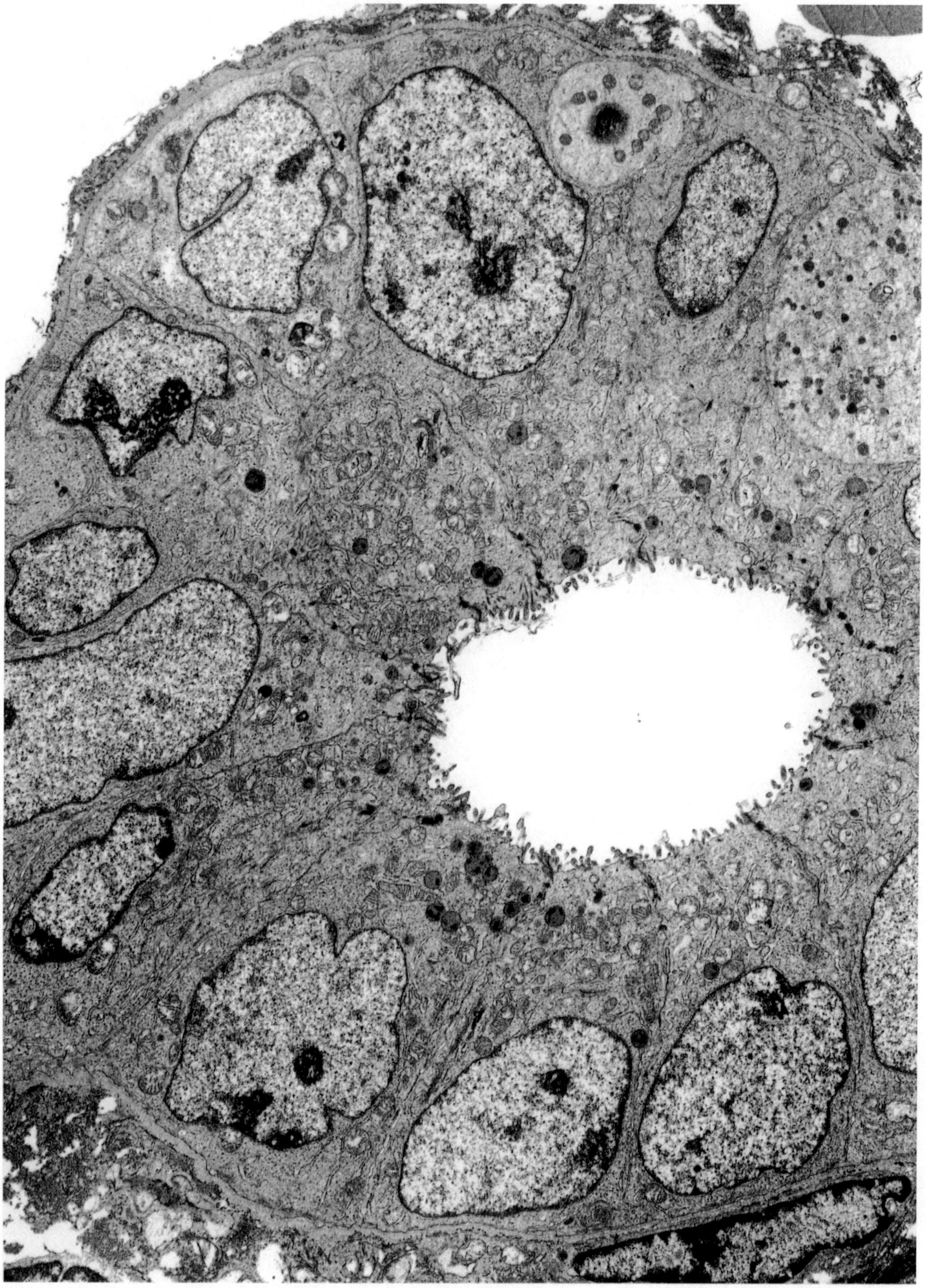

3 Pancreatitis

3.1 Definition and Classification

Inflammatory diseases of the pancreas are characterized by autodigestion of the gland by the enzymes produced by itself. It is therefore referred to as autodigestive-tryptic pancreatitis. Less frequently uncharacteristic or ordinary interstitial pancreatitis as a concomitant reaction to general diseases can be observed aside from this, in which signs of autodigestion are missing. Both varieties can take their course as acute, or acute or chronic recurring reactions. The ordinary variety of pancreatitis can transgress to an autodigestive or a chronic progressive variety at any time (Remmele 1984).

Inspite of many attempts a generally acknowledged and valid classification of pancreatitis, which takes both clinical symptoms and histomorphological findings equally into consideration, has not yet been introduced.

The classification based especially on the clinical aspects in respect to the therapeutic approach, developed at the symposium at Marseille in 1963 (Sarles 1965), was revised in 1984 (Singer 1985) and is acknowledged as the general foundation of the classification of the disease today. Accordingly an acute and chronic pancreatitis are distinguished from one another (Table 2). The acute variety can take its course in singular or intermittent episodes. Complete restoration of health is possible in this type, whereas a progressive course is generally observed in chronic pancreatitis. It too, can take its course in singular or intermittent episodes.

Clinical experience acknowledges the weaknesses of this classification, which is correct by systematic-classifactory aspects. Distinguishing between an episode of acute, relapsing pancreatitis and an acute episode of chronic pancreatitis is often impossible, even with modern diagnostic methods. The designation of an inflammatory episode as an acute or chronic variety of the disease can only be performed catamnestically in most cases.

In the discussion surrounding the new Marseille Classification (Singer 1985) it was established that pseudocysts in acute pancreatitis are considered a persistent defect after healing and not a sign of transgression to a chronic course of the inflammatory disease. Permanent residual damage with development of pseudocysts does, however, occur in chronic pancreatitis (Volkholz and Stolte 1984, Singer 1985).

Table 2 Classification of pancreatitis according to the Marseille nomenclature of 1963 (Sarles, 1965)

Types	Characteristics	Course
acute pancreatitis	single episode	cure possible
acute, relapsing pancreatitis	several episodes	
chronic pancreatitis	non episodal	
chronic, relapsing pancreatitis	several episodes	progressive

Table 3 Classification of pancreatitis according to the revised Marseille nomenclature of 1984 (Singer, 1985)

Types	Characteristics	Course
acute pancreatitis	single episode or several episodes	cure possible
chronic pancreatitis	single episode or several episodes	progressive

Abscess formation in the pancreas is based on secondary infection of a primarily aseptic necrosis. It is more frequently a complication of acute pancreatitis and much more infrequently does it occur in an acute episode of chronic pancreatitis. An abscess can also develop in a pseudocyst with secondary infection.

Already upon introduction of the classification it was ascertained that the degree of severity of the clinical course of acute pancreatitis can not be correlated with the pathologic-anatomic findings in many cases. Furthermore, because of the uncertainty in establishing the causal relationship designation of pancreatitis to etiological factors was dispensed with.

3.2 Etiology of Pancreatitis (Fig. 18)

Inspite of intense endeavors the etiology and pathogenesis of pancreatitis have not been sufficiently identified (Creutzfeld 1987). Biliary causes in 40 to 80% and chronic alcohol abuse in approximately 30% of the cases are alleged to be the most frequent etiological factors involved in the development of pancreatitis (Rösch 1983, Phat et al. 1984). Other components are also topics of discussion, but they are understood as rare causes (Table 4).

The frequency of the etiologies in individual statistical synopses is dependent on the age distribution of the patients. Alcohol abuse is a more frequent cause of the disease in young men, whereas in older women bile duct afflictions generally are the causal agent of pancreatitis.

Stone impaction in close proximity to the papilla, however, is found only in 2 to 5% of the cases, whereas cholelithiasis is present in 20% of the cases. In the majority of patients biliary calculi are found in the stool (Acosta and Ledesma 1974). In individual cases it remains difficult to ascertain which pathogenetic role cholelithiasis played in the development of pancreatitis. Clinical experience has indicated that surgical revision of the bile ducts prevents relapses of pancreatitis (Howard and Jordan 1956, Hollender et al. 1983).

Individual duct anatomy is of crucial significance in biliary reflux pancreatitis. The various course-, tributary- and orificial variants of the ducts of Wirsung, Santorini and Choledochus as well as the ab-

Table 4 Etiological factors of tryptic haemorrhagic pancreatitis

- Cholelithiasis and other biliary causes
- Alcohol abuse
- Drugs, e.g. steroids
- Toxins, e.g. E 605
- Uraemia
- Metabolic acidosis
- Hyperparathyroidism
- Protein deficiency
- Hormonal disturbances e.g. gestational pancreatitis
- Hyperlipemia, especially Fredrikson's Type V
- Immunological factors, e.g. lupus erythematodes
- Neural factors, e.g. excessive vagal stimulation
- Circulatory disturbances
- Infectious causes

(Becker, 1984, Dammann, 1981, Remmele, 1984)

Fig. 18
Obstruction of the main bile duct and pancreatic duct as a cause of an acute necrotizing pancreatitis. Autopsy situs. Cholelithiasis. Impacted stone in the common final stretch between the common bile and pancreatic ducts directly before the papilla of Vateri (arrow 1). Bile reflux into the pancreatic duct with green discoloration of the ductal mucosa (arrow 2). Extensively confluent necrosis of the pancreatic head (arrow 3).

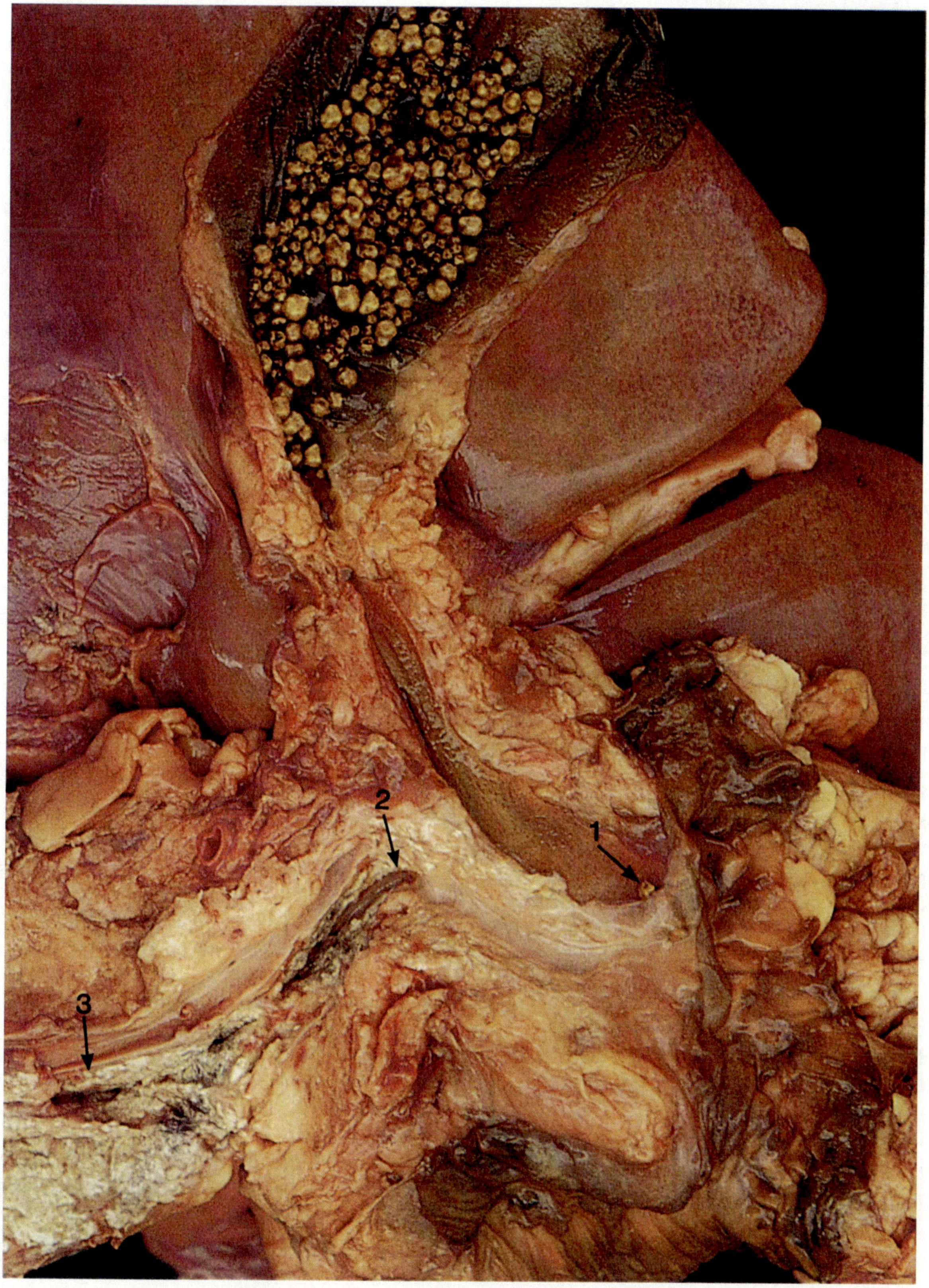
2
1
3

sence of accessory salivary duct orifices in the common bile duct determine the morphologic picture and the intrapancreatic distribution pattern of biliary pancreatitis. It is remarkable with which frequency the occurrence of idiopathic acute pancreatitis without any recognizable cause, on an average in 39% of the cases, is reported (Goebbel 1980, Roggenwallner 1985).

Friedrich (1878) and Fitz (1889) already recognized the connection between advanced pancreatic diseases and alcoholism and coined the term "drinker's pancreatitis".

The occurrence of alcohol-induced pancreatitis (potatory pancreatitis, pancreatitis subsequent to an opulent meal) in the statistics is misleading. It can be maintained that in most cases an acute episode of an already chronic pancreatitis occurs and thus only an acute phase of an essentially progressive disease of the pancreas takes place.

After 8 to 10 years of an average consumption of 80 to 120g of alcohol per day inflammation of the pancreas occurs frequently (Becker 1984). The pathogenetic principle of the effect of alcohol on the pancreas has remained obscure heretofore inspite of a great number of experimental investigations, some of the findings also being contradictory.

A direct toxic effect on the pancreatic parenchymal cells analagous to the effect on hepatic parenchymal cells and a functional disturbance of the gland to the effect of dyschylia are alleged to be triggering causes of alcohol-induced pancreatitis (Rösch 1983). Metaplastic and proliferative alterations of the ductal epithelium and fatty degeneration of the acinar cells are considered to be indications of toxic damage (Remmele 1984).

In the pancreas damaged by alcohol increased protein and protein precipitates can be frequently demonstrated in the efferent ducts. This alteration is interpreted as a function-increasing effect due to increased cholecystokinin-secretion following alcohol-induced alteration of the parasympathetic tonus (Remmele 1984).

According to other studies the toxic damage to the ductal epithelium is claimed to be the cause of inflammation. The missing influence of secretin on the damaged ductal epithelium leads to a decrease in water and electrolyte efflux via the ductal epithelium. The protein precipitates in the lumina of the ducts would thus not be the result of absolute proteochylia due to an increase in protein secretion but of deficient dilution of the secreted proteins due to decreased water- and electrolyte output (Remmele 1984).

Aside from the direct effect of alcohol on the epithelial constituents of the pancreas indirect effects are also maintained. In the course of alcohol-induced gastroduodenitis a spasm of Oddi's sphincter can be evoked, causing congestion in the pancreas similar to that caused by occlusion of the duct in stone impaction. Increased pressure in the duodenum in gastroduodenitis with reflux of duodenal contents into the pancreatic duct can possibly be the cause of inflammation (Dürr 1978).

Although the etiology and the pathogenesis of pancreatitis has not been completely solved it can be maintained that the autodigestion occurring by activation of proenzymes prior to their reaching the intestinal lumen is of vital importance (Creutzfeld 1987). The primary process initiating the so-called "pancreatic enzyme cascade" (Rinderknecht 1986) is the activation of trypsinogen to trypsin. Trypsin activates the other zymogens, especially phospholipase A, which liberates the aggressive lysolecithin from lecithin. Until now it has been generally believed that the activation of small amounts of trypsin must occur extracellularly. Experimental studies have shown, however, that probably under the influence of lysosomal enzymes intracellular activation can take place (Rao et al. 1980).

The enzymes produced and secreted in the pancreas can maintain the inflammation. By means of proteolysis trypsin and chymotrypsin give rise to oedema and coagulation necrosis with haemorrhagia due to direct alteration of the vascular walls. Elastase is involved in the vascular alterations by causing lysis of the elastic fibres. Kallikrein elicits liberation of kallidin, which attacks the vascular walls and can lead to shock symptoms. Phospholipase A and lipase, which are activated by bile acids, maintain the tissue necrosis by producing lysophospholipids. Pancreatic lipase cleaves triglycerides and leads to characteristic fat necroses (Remmele 1984).

Postoperative acute pancreatitis can occur particularly after upper abdominal operations. The clinical picture is rare. The frequency claimed in the literature is variable. Following transduodenal papillotomy a frequency of 4% was determined, following gastric resection percentages ranging from 0.5 to 1.5% were calculated. According to these studies Billroth II gastric resections show a higher disposition to pancreatitis than Billroth I gastroduodenal anastomoses (Bünte 1971). Every operation involving the pancreas itself, including a biopsy, can lead to postoperative pancreatitis.

Intraoperative endoscopic examinations of the bile and pancreatic ducts or the performance of an ERCP can elicit an acute inflammatory reaction even in a not previously damaged pancreas. The increased injection pressure exceeding 50 to 70 cm water column is mainly responsible for this (Mallet-Guy et al. 1957). Postoperative pancreatitis is rare, but its overall prognosis is bad. It is alleged to have a 40% lethality (Farthmann and Männl 1980, Bünte 1971).

Drug-induced acute pancreatitis, e.g. by thiazides or following application of glucocorticoids, is not so rare. Lindner (1964) reported 6 deaths due to acute pancreatitis in 115 patients with cirrhosis of the liver, who had been treated with prednisolone. Long-term medication with corticosteroids intervenes in the structural and functional metabolism of the acinar cells and a type of dyschylia can ensue (Hollender et al. 1983).

3.3 Acute Pancreatitis (Figs. 18–48)

3.3.1 Definition

Acute pancreatitis is an episodal inflammation which can occur as a disease in its own right or concomitantly during another primary disease. It can heal completely with a restitutio ad integrum or it can transgress to a haemorrhagic-necrotizing variety and in turn, lead to serious, life endangering symptoms.

3.3.2 Clinical Course

The clinical course of acute pancreatitis is characterized by a downright brutal onset "out of the blue" (Hentschel 1978). At the beginning of the disease the cardinal symptom is pain. It can elicit infarction-like pain and incapacitating distress. The boring pain in the upper abdomen can radiate in a belt-like manner to the back via the right and left flanks. The patient lies in a "prayer position" (Hollender et al. 1983). The pain spreads quickly to the complete abdomen. The actual attack rarely occurs out of complete health. In about 60% of the cases slight attacks of pain in the upper abdomen had been experienced previously (Hess 1969). Nausea, vomiting and an ileus are often secondary to the extreme state of pain which occasionally can hardly be controlled by analgesics. There is abdominal muscle rigidity, which compared to the abdominal muscle rigidity occurring initially upon perforation of a hollow organ with consecutive peritonitis is not "stone hard", but equals an abdominal resistance of more elastic consistency. Creutzfeld (1977) coined the expression "rubber stomach".

In serious cases signs of shock with hypotension, tachycardia and cold sweat present as the major symptoms. In other cases there is conspicuous facial redness (rubeosis), probably as an indication of an enzymatical vascular paralysis (Hess 1969). Occasionally the dramatic course leads to a rapid decline of the patient within hours.

Already in initial stages paralytic ileus is present, involving only the duodenum and jejunum to begin with, affecting further parts of the intestine later, in particular the colon. It is caused by in part extensive fat necroses in the mesenterium and venous congestion of the bowel. Aside from intestinal paralysis, ascites can be revealed by percussion even on the first day (Bohnsack et al. 1983).

Various alterations of the skin, occurring only in approximately 10% of the cases, however, can be observed. Prognostic significance is attributed to so-called "Warren's" or "Cullen's sign". It is blue discoloration around the umbilicus resulting from oedematous infiltration. Early appearance of the sign supposedly indicates massive pancreatic damage and thus a bad prognosis.

In approximately 40% of the cases pleural effusions develop in the course of the disease. They are most frequently found on the left side, often bilateral and not infrequently combined with pericardial effusion. According to the composition it is an exudate with increased amylase content.

Liberation of the active pancreatic enzymes via the blood, lymphatics and ascites can lead to severe alterations in the liver, kidneys and lung (Stömmer 1987). A shock-induced drop in blood pressure, activated tissue hormones and haemo- and myolysis can lead to acute renal failure. The kidneys are enlarged and exhibit tubulonephrosis or -necrosis. Haemoglobin, myoglobin and erythrocyte cylinders can be demonstrated in the lumina of the tubules. Occasionally the capillaries of the glomerula are occluded by thrombi.

A serious complication of tryptic pancreatitis is acute lung failure. The frequency is dependent on the severity of the acute pancreatitis and according to clinical investigations occurs in a frequency up to 73% of the cases. Ischaemic alterations of the retina in acute pancreatitis have been reported. Fat embolism or rather aggregates of granulocytes were considered causal agents (Hollender et al. 1983).

Complications involving the central nervous system occur in 9 to 19% of the cases (Colmant and Noltenius 1977). Delirious, hallucinatory and paranoid states and disturbances of consciousness up to comatose states occur. These symptoms represent shock-induced central venous damage. Furthermore a remote toxic effect of the pancreatic enzymes are topic of discussion.

Pancreatic encephalopathy forms an independent symptom complex and is not related to chronic alcohol abuse, as it also occurs in non-alcoholic patients. In about 10 to 20% of the patients with severe acute pancreatitis an increased convulsive potential can be observed.

Subcutaneous "metastatic" fat necroses may be found less frequently. Indurated, painful, occasionally haemorrhagic nodules arise. The fat necroses may occur in the thoracic wall, the buttocks, particularly in the retroperitoneum and the renal capsules (Hess 1969).

3.3.3 Diagnostics (Figs. 19–25)

Extreme upper abdominal pain, nausea, emesis and abdominal rigidity characterize the clinical picture of acute pancreatitis. Not all cases of pancreatitis take a typical course and can be distinguished from other acute abdominal disorders without further studies. Atypical courses of the disease are relatively frequent.

The following diagnostic measures are necessary to establish two complexes:

1. Verification or improbability of the suspected diagnosis
2. Assessment of the severity of the disease for determination of the radius of necessary therapeutic measures.

Determining the severity of the disease was a special problem for a long time because of the topographic situation of the organ.

Principally the diagnostics of diseases of parenchymatous organs are based on clinico-chemical examination methods, endoscopic diagnostics and visual aids including x-ray diagnostics. Additionally diagnostic laparotomy is available as a last resort. Of the clinico-chemical examination methods determining the alpha-amylase and lipase levels are of particular practical significance. Determination of the lipase levels always increases the diagnostic yield as it occurs only in the pancreas. False positive findings are not infrequent. Thus in more than half of the diagnostic ERCP an elevation of amylase exists without pancreatitis present in nearly that frequency (Büchler et al. 1985).

Most conventional radiological methods have yielded disappointing results with respect to patient observation, management and determining the severity of the acute pancreatitis. Pancreatic scintigraphy involves a high radiation dose and is neither very sensitive nor specific (Bücheler et al. 1985).

ERCP is contraindicated in acute pancreatitis because of the considerable risk of aggravating the course of the disease. Plain x-ray films of the abdomen and upper gastrointestinal x-rays with barium studies offer too few details as to the severity of the pancreatitis.

Newer diagnostic visual methods such as sonography and computerized tomography (CT) have recently gained special significance in patient observation and assessment of the degree of severity of acute pancreatitis. Upper abdominal sonography is a quick, riskless, stressless investigation method, which is thus especially suitable for sequential studies. It is characterized by a very high diagnostic yield (Lackner et al. 1980). Cholecysto-choledocholithiasis, one of the most important

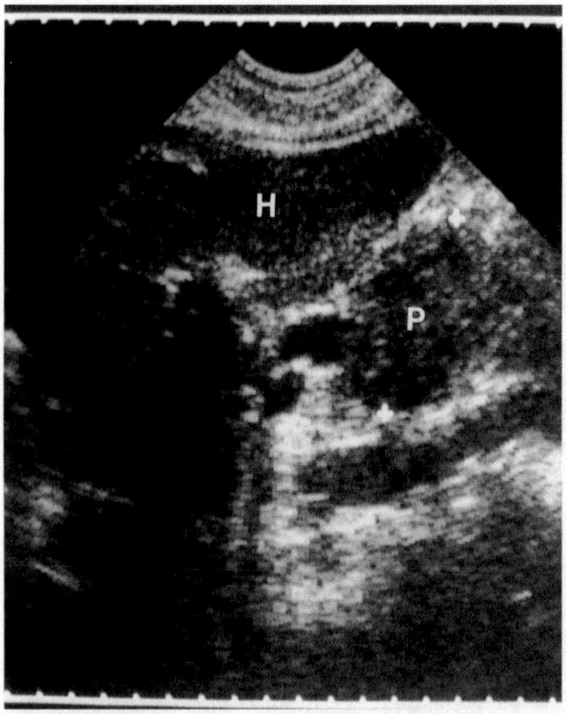

Fig. 19
Sonographic findings in acute necrotizing pancreatitis. Extensive necrosis of the pancreatic head (P). Contours of the liver recognizable above (H).

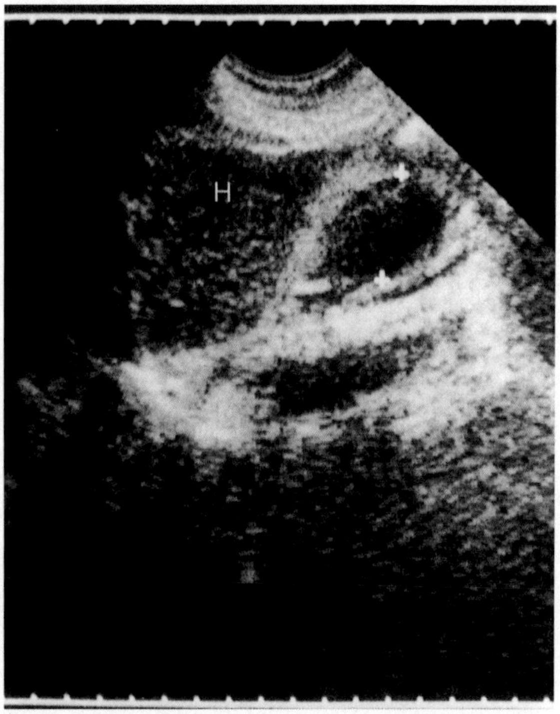

Fig. 20
Sonographic longitudinal section depicting a pancreatic cyst (between the crosses). Adjacent shadow of the liver (H).

causal pathogenetic factors can be demonstrated by sonography in more than 90% of the cases.

Like sonography, computerized tomography (CT) contributes to the detection of etiological factors leading to verification of the diagnosis, assessment of the severity of the disease and detection of complications. Advantages and disadvantages of this method are summarized in Table 5.

To establish the diagnosis of pancreatitis the following approach is indicated: Sonography should be performed to distinguish the diagnosis from other upper abdominal disorders and to search for a biliary cause. Pancreatic oedema requires close sequential sonographic controls. If in sonography suspicion arises that acute haemorrhagic-necrotizing pancreatitis is present, computerized tomography is indicated, especially if surgical interven-

Table 5 Advantages and disadvantages of sonography and computerized tomography (Lackner et al. 1980)

Advantages of sonography	Disadvantages of sonography
1. Variable direction of sectioning 2. Differentiation of solid and liquid structures 3. Registration of dynamic parameters 4. Bedside examination of the patients 5. No risk examination 6. No radiation load 7. Low examination costs	1. Picture trouble due to great variations in oscillations 2. Penetration of sound waves is limited 3. Examination of patients recently operated on is often not possible 4. Picture quality often dependent on experience of the examiner
Advantages of computerized tomography	**Disadvantages of computerized tomography**
1. Extensive anatomic-topographic overview 2. Registration of parenchymal densities 3. Functional diagnostics subsequent to i.v. contrast medium application 4. Broad spectrum of application 5. Standard recording technique 6. Easy interpretation of picture contents 7. No disturbance by superimposition of skeletal parts or gaseous intestinal contents	1. Artefacts due to movements of uncooperative patients 2. Bad dissolution of organs in extremely lean patients 3. High costs

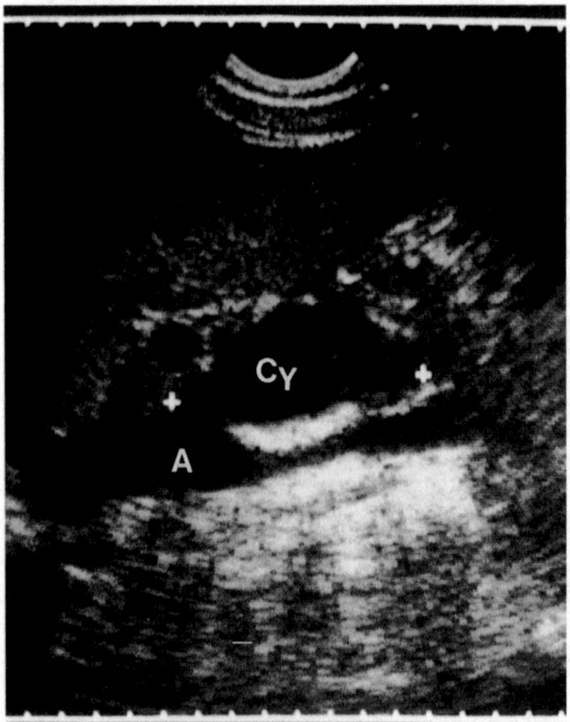

Fig. 21
Sonographic longitudinal section localizing a cyst (cy) below the liver and on the aorta (a).

tion is being considered. The extent of necroses and the proportion of the necrotizing process beyond the pancreas (necrosis channels) can be assessed. Based on the findings of the CT-scan as a reference, sequential sonographic controls must be performed (Neher et al. 1982).

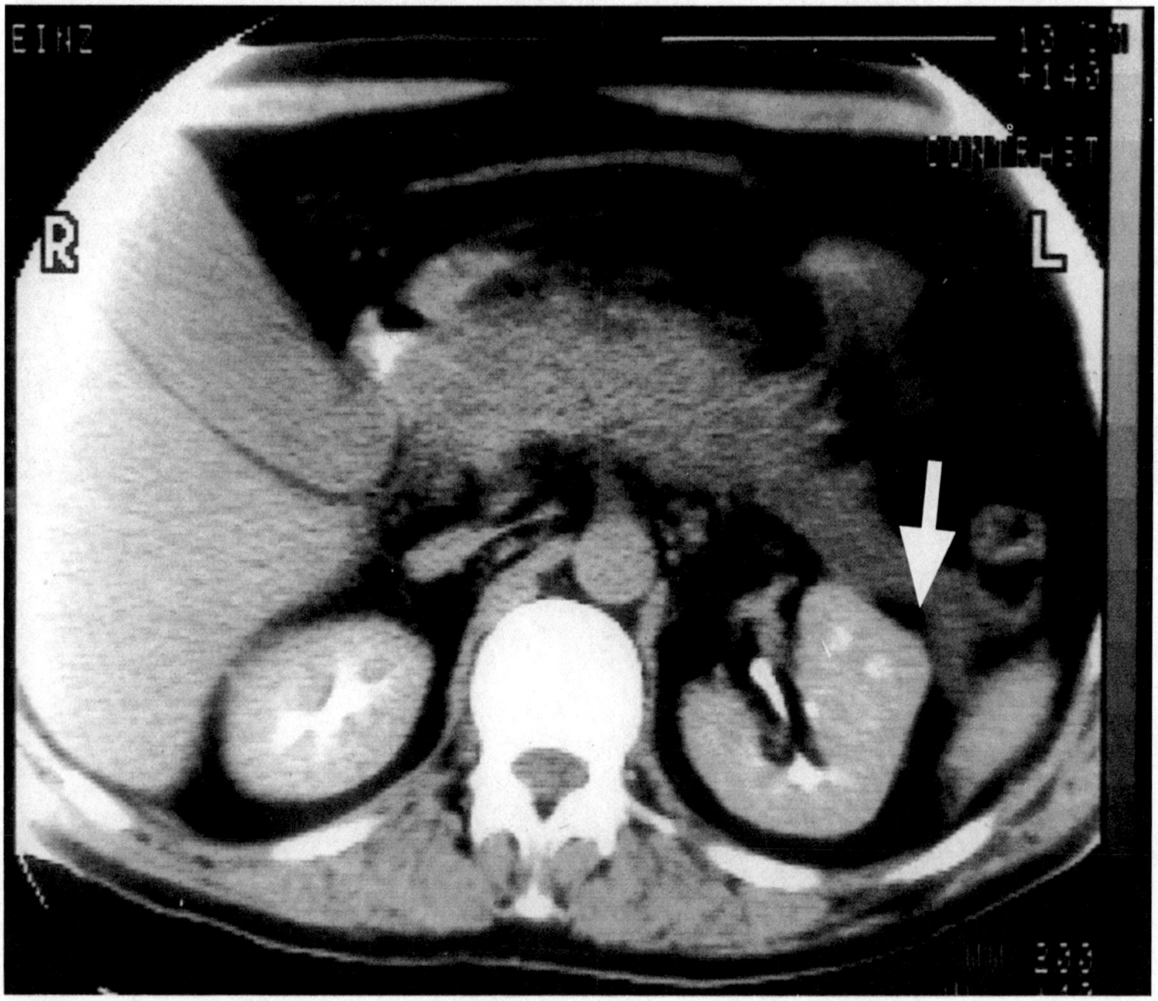

Fig. 22
Computerized tomograph. Acute necrotizing pancreatitis with retroperitoneal channel of necrosis (arrow).

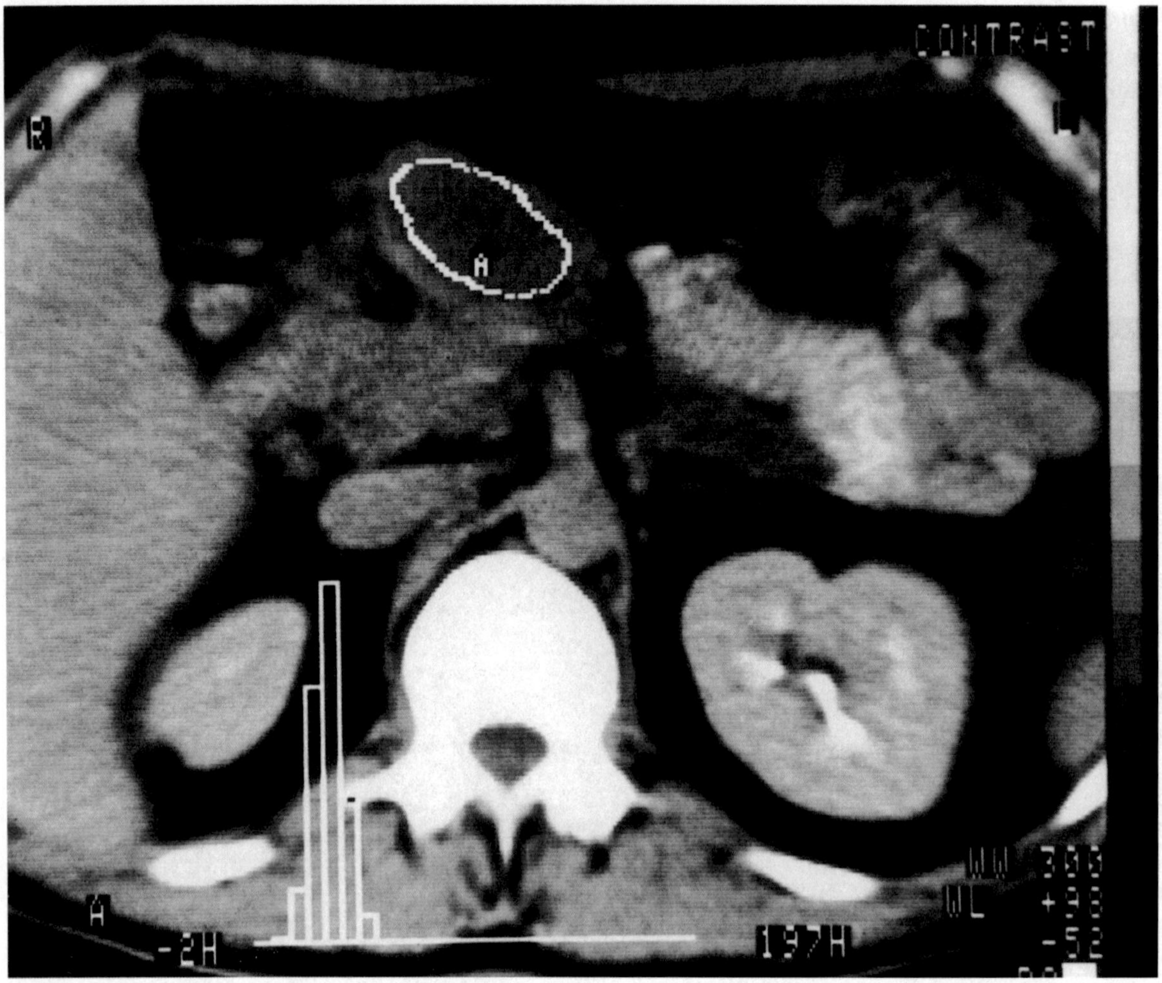

Fig. 23
Computerized tomograph. Acute necrotizing pancreatitis with abscess formation in the uncinate process (marked by dotted line).

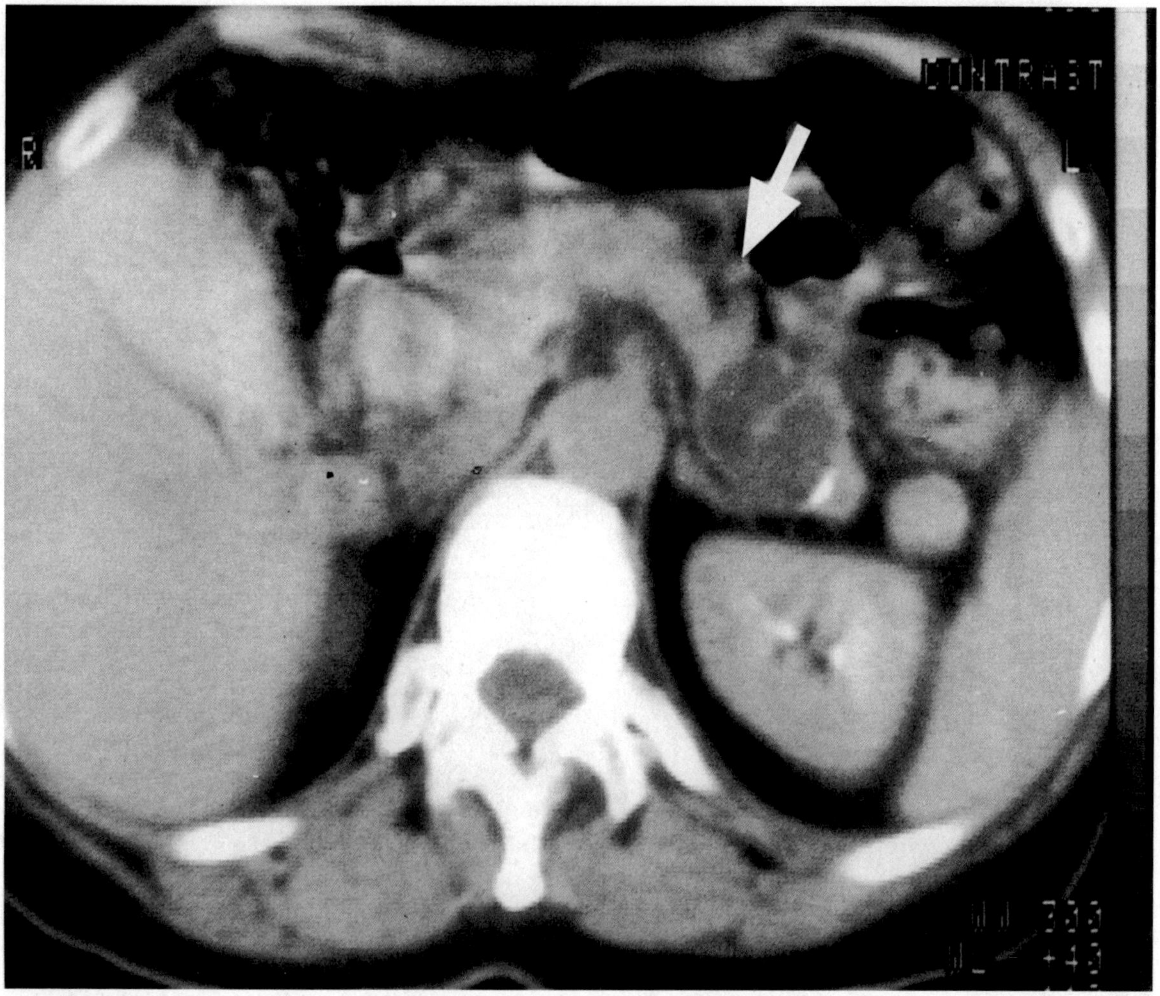

Fig. 24
Computerized tomograph. Acute necrotizing pancreatitis with abscess formation in the pancreatic tail (arrow).

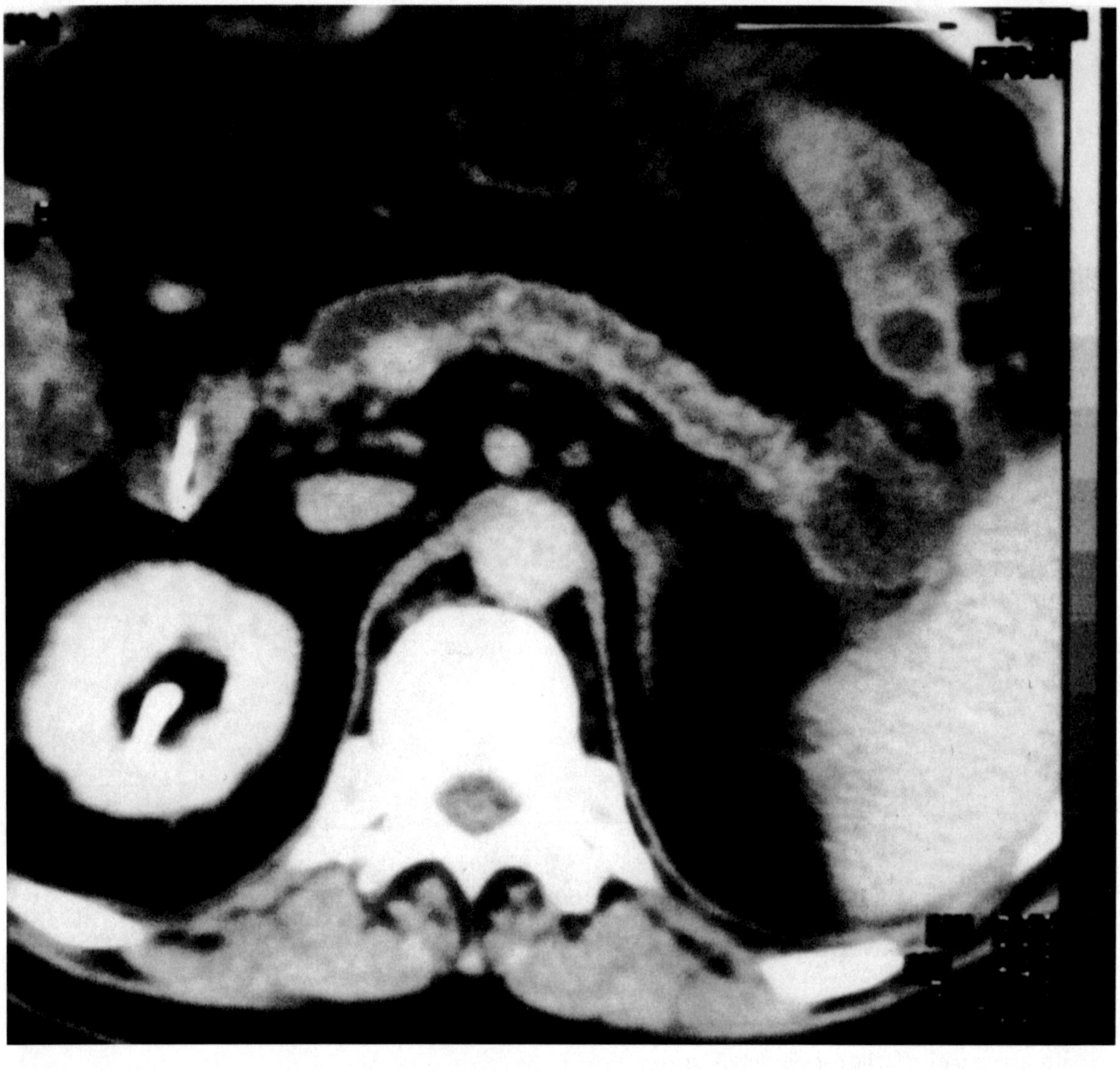

Fig. 25
Computerized tomograph. Acute necrotizing pancreatitis. The structure of the organ is hardly discernable. Parts of the duct of Wirsung are still intact.

3.3.4 Prognosis of Acute Pancreatitis

The course of the disease and its prognosis depend considerably on the severity of the disease. In recent years a grading of the severity of pancreatitis has become generally accepted.

When oedematous pancreatitis (Grade I) occurs, there is
- no icterus
- no severe deviations in the following parameters: blood glucose, serum calcium, creatinine and haematocrit

Grade II (limited pancreatic necrosis) is characterized by:
- subicterus
- severe alterations of the following parameters to some extent: blood glucose, serum calcium, creatinine and haematocrit
- progressive deterioration inspite of conservative intensive care

Grade III (diffuse necrotizing pancreatitis) is characterized by:
- respiratory failure, encephalopathy
- severe alterations of the following parameters: blood glucose, serum calcium, creatinine and haematocrit
- progressive deterioration inspite of conservative intensive care

Whereas in oedematous pancreatitis hardly any deaths occur, the lethality rate increases steeply up to III. grade pancreatitis. Death rates of 80 % and more inspite of combined conservative and surgical treatment are not a rarity. It thus becomes obvious that earliest diagnosis possible determines the rate of success in the treatment of II. and III. grade pancreatitis. Several authors have tried to determine reliable parameters enabling differentiation of the different forms of pancreatitis (Table 6).

Dammann and Grabbe (1981) have tried to include clinical results as well as computerized tomographic findings in their grading. Depending on the percentual distribution of the individual parameters in the deceased they interpret these criteria differently. On the basis of their results they distinguish between severe and mild courses of acute pancreatitis.

Table 6 Ranson's unfavorable prognostic parameters in acute pancreatitis (1978) revised by Hollender et al. (1983)

Early findings
Age higher than 55 years
Serum glucose exceeding 200 mg/dl
Leucocytosis exceeding 16000/Mikro I
LDH exceeding 350 U/l
Control findings (24–48 hours after onset of illness)
Reduction in haematocrit by more than 10%
Serum calcium concentration lower than 2.0 mmol/l
Base deficit higher than 4.0 mmol/l
Arterial pO_2 lower than 60 mm Hg
Fluid deficit more than 6 l

Agreement has not been reached as to the significance of the parameters determining the prognosis. It is pointed out in a different context, that the parameters "GOT" and "leucocytosis" mentioned as particularly relevant in Ranson's synopsis, are of no or only subordinate prognostic significance (Dammann and Döpner 1981). The uncertainty still existing in respect to assessment of the degree of severity of the disease is responsible for the uncertainty in determining the right moment for adequate therapeutic measures, especially for surgical intervention, if it proves necessary. Undoubtedly surgical intervention is necessary prior to manifestation of organ complications, as the prognosis deteriorates dramatically upon their onset (Klose et al. 1983).

In this connection Hoefler (1979) states that the optimal moment for surgery is the time span between the 5. and 7. day of illness. He argues this on the grounds that in this period of time the lethality due to kinogenic shock as well as early intoxications (in his collective of patients 57.6%) from byproducts of protein metabolism decreases. After the 7. day of illness a 2. crisis arises, often with irreparable organ complications. This 2. crisis can be prevented by surgical intervention. Schuster et al. (1980) point out the so-called "lethal triad" and define it as acute renal and respiratory failure in haemorrhagic-necrotizing pancreatitis. In this state any therapeutic measures are generally too late. By early surgical intervention to remove the focus of primary disease the lethal triad can be prevented. Schuster et al. (1980) speak of the significance of sepsis as a crucial complication in the course of the disease, which in turn can call forth further organ complications. In the literature shock and heart failure are alleged to be the most frequent cause of death. Infections, liver and renal failure as well as haemorrhages and pulmonary embolism can also be causes of death.

3.3.5 Morphology of Acute Pancreatitis (Figs. 18, 26–48)

3.3.5.1 Gross Findings (Fig. 18)

From the morphologic findings acute pancreatitis can be classified by severity into three grades. Oedematous pancreatitis corresponds with grade I. The capsule is intact, the contours of the lobuli are prominent. The alterations are confined to the glands. The capsule is strained. On palpation the organ is bouncy. The surface of the cut is mottled.

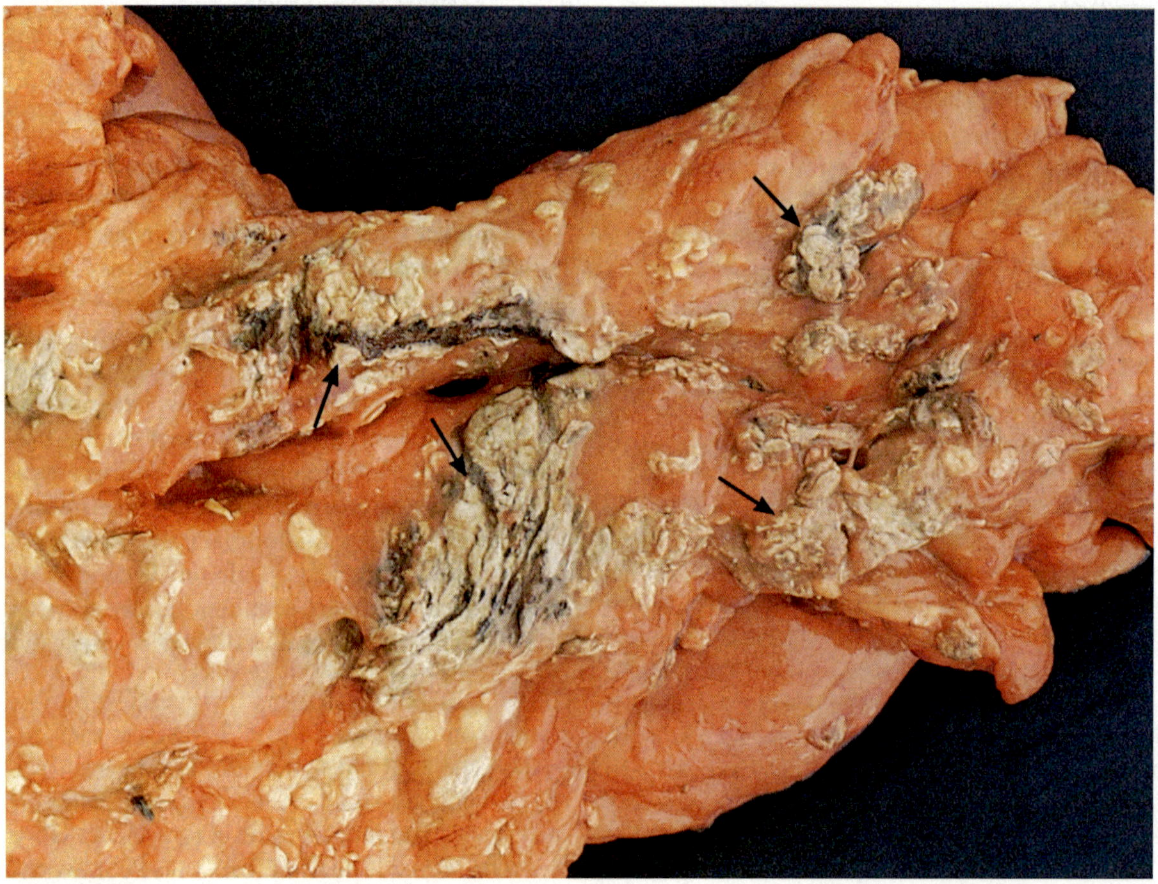

Fig. 26
Gross alterations in acute pancreatitis Grade I. The capsule is intact. The lobular outlines are distinct. At the surface of the cut adjacent to haemorrhagic zones of necrosis (arrows) relatively altered parenchyma

Aside from haemorrhagic zones of necrosis there can be unaltered areas. Hyperaemic and anaemic areas can occur next to one another. In the subcapsular fatty tissue scattered fat necroses can be developed.

In grade II necrosis is more extensive and fat necrosis can be demonstrated in the rest of the abdominal cavity even though the rest of the capsule is still intact. The gland is greatly enlarged and shows a distinct border to the neighboring organs. The consistency is hard as stone. The cutting surface is of a dark red colour. The border between necrotic and intact glandular areas cannot be exactly defined. The contours of the lobuli become indistinct. The necroses extend to the periductal glandular tissue. The necroses are variably haemorrhagic.

Total necrosis of the organ characterizes grade III. The borders of the organ are no longer distinct. The necroses extend to neighboring organs. Fat

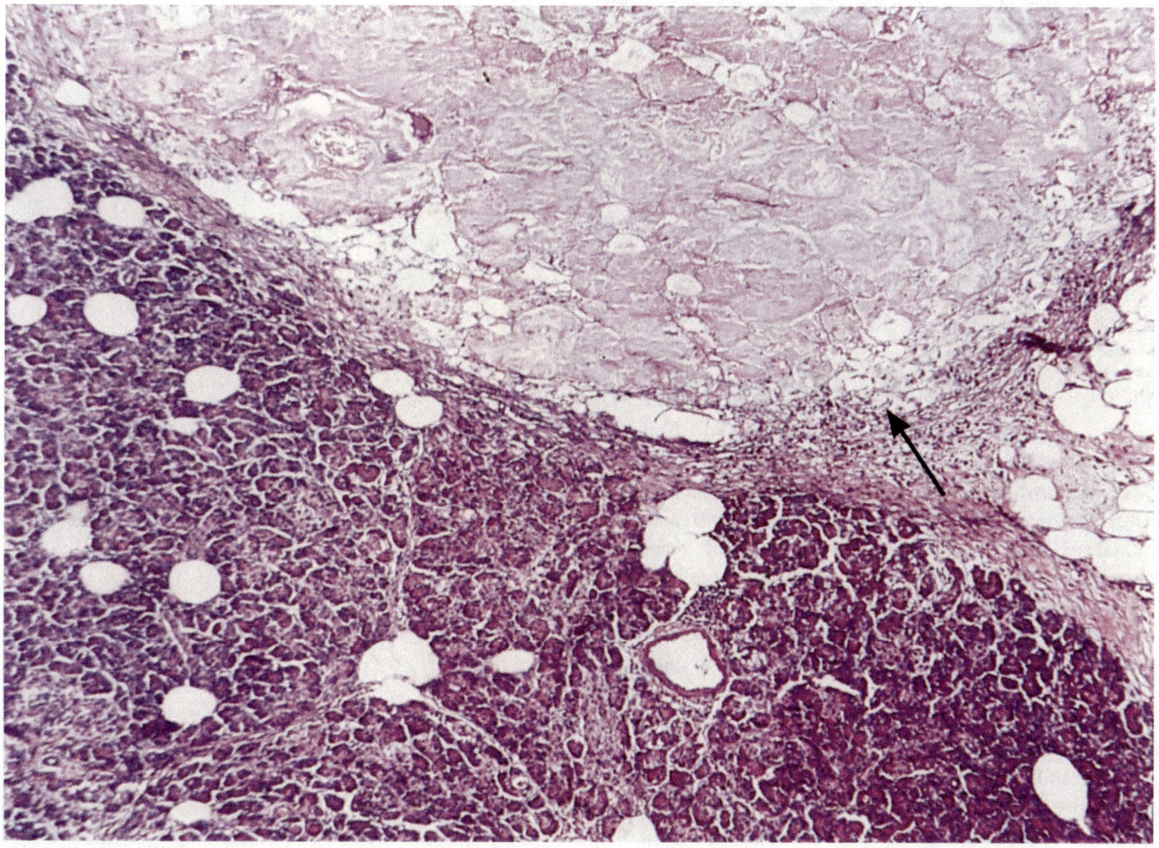

Fig. 27
Oedematous pancreatitis. Oedematous imbibition of the acinar structure without alteration of the individual epithelial components. Only scattered, well-circumscribed fat necroses (arrow) can be demonstrated.
Light micrograph
Stain:hematoxylin:eosin
Magnification: 95 ×

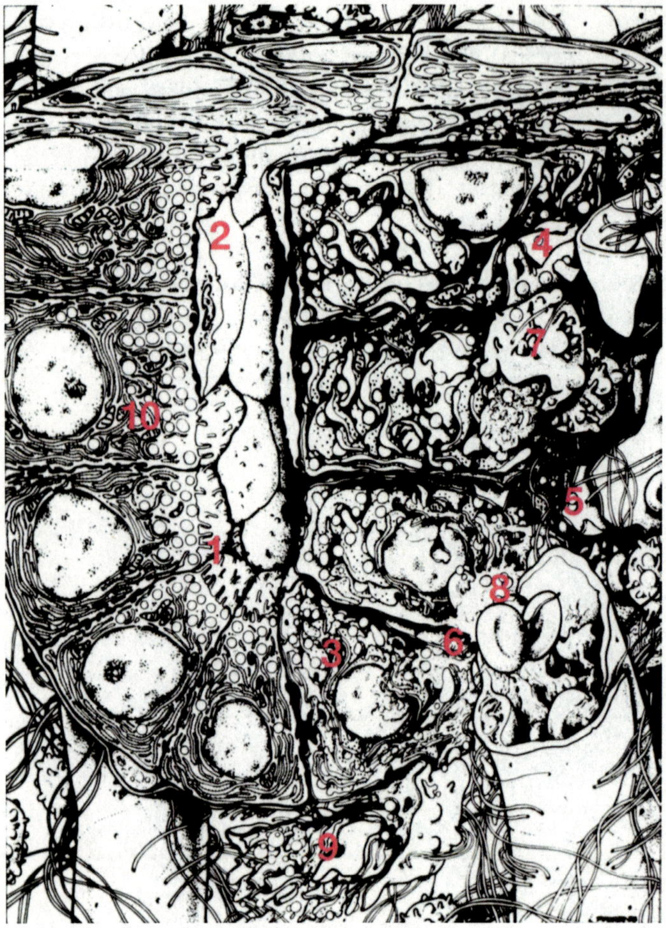

Fig. 28
Three-dimensional reconstruction. Alterations of the acinar epithelial cells in acute necrotizing pancreatitis. Intracellular oedema of individual epithelial cells with vesicular distension of the endoplasmic reticulum. Irregularly arranged zymogen granula and release of the granula into the interstitial connective tissue. Dissolution of the membrane system of the cells. Extension of the necrosis to the capillary walls.

1. acinar lumen
2. centro-acinar cells
3. intracellular oedema of the acinar cells
4. opening of the basal cell membrane
5. Release of zymogen granula into the interstitium
6. Distension of the intercellular spaces
7. macrophages
8. Necrosis of the capillary wall with haemorrhage
9. Mast cell with liberation of granula
10. Intact acinar cells

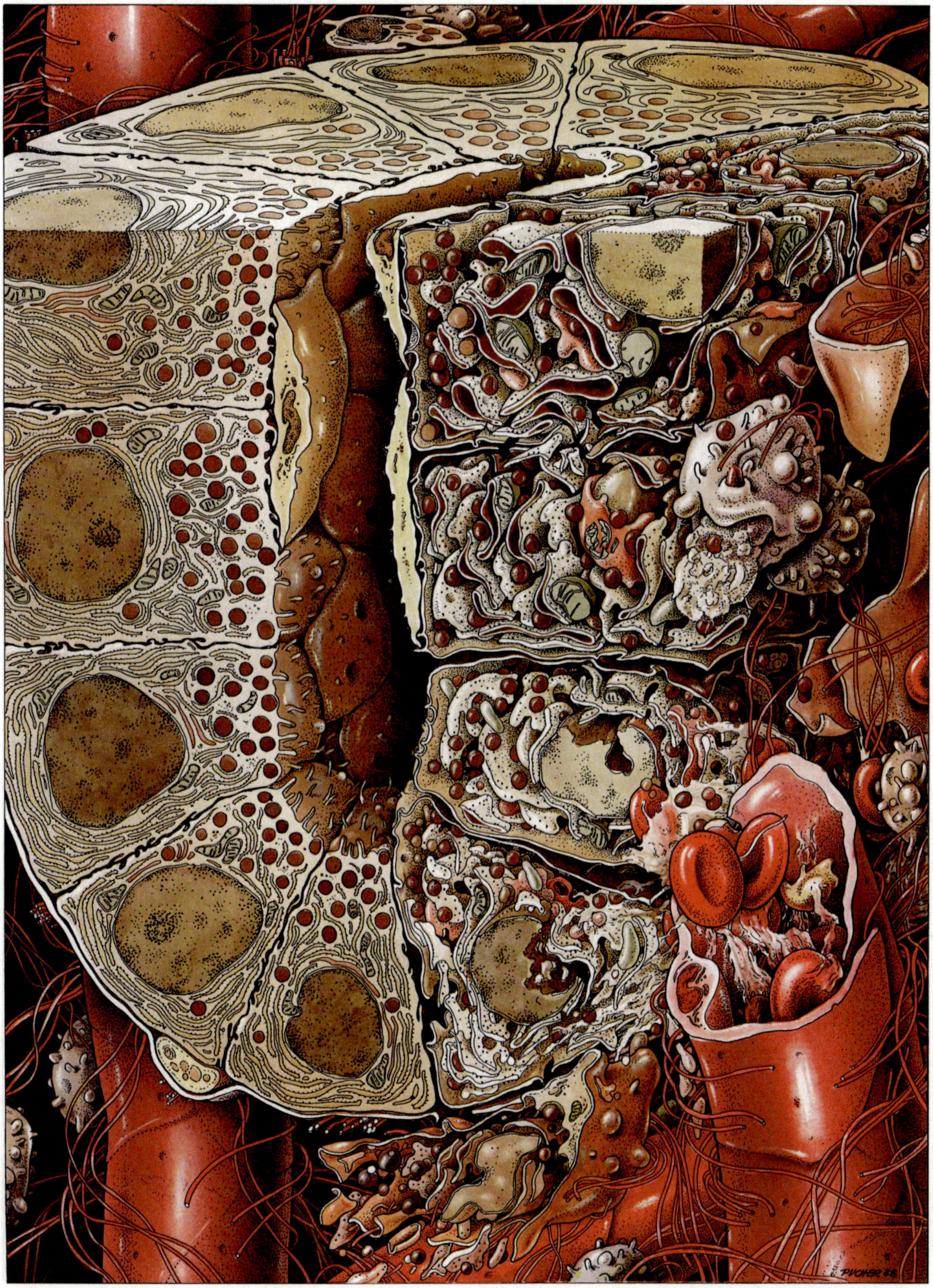

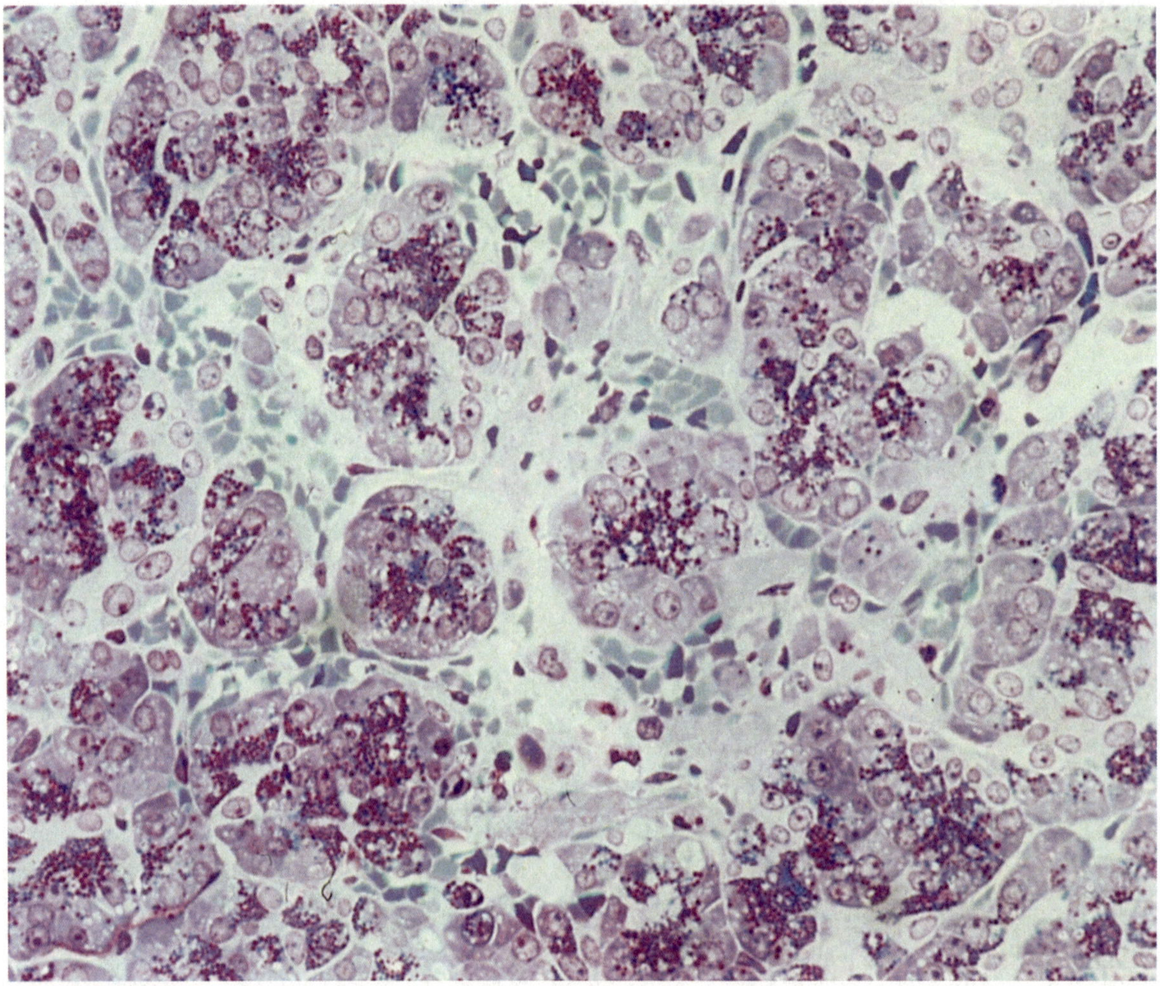

Fig. 29
Acute necrotizing pancreatitis. Intercellular oedema with dispersion of the acinar structure. In intact acini irregular secretory activity in individual epithelial cells. Marked dilatation of the capillaries and hyperaemia.
Light micrograph
Semithin section
Stain: Basic fuchsin and methylene blue.
Magnification: 380 ×

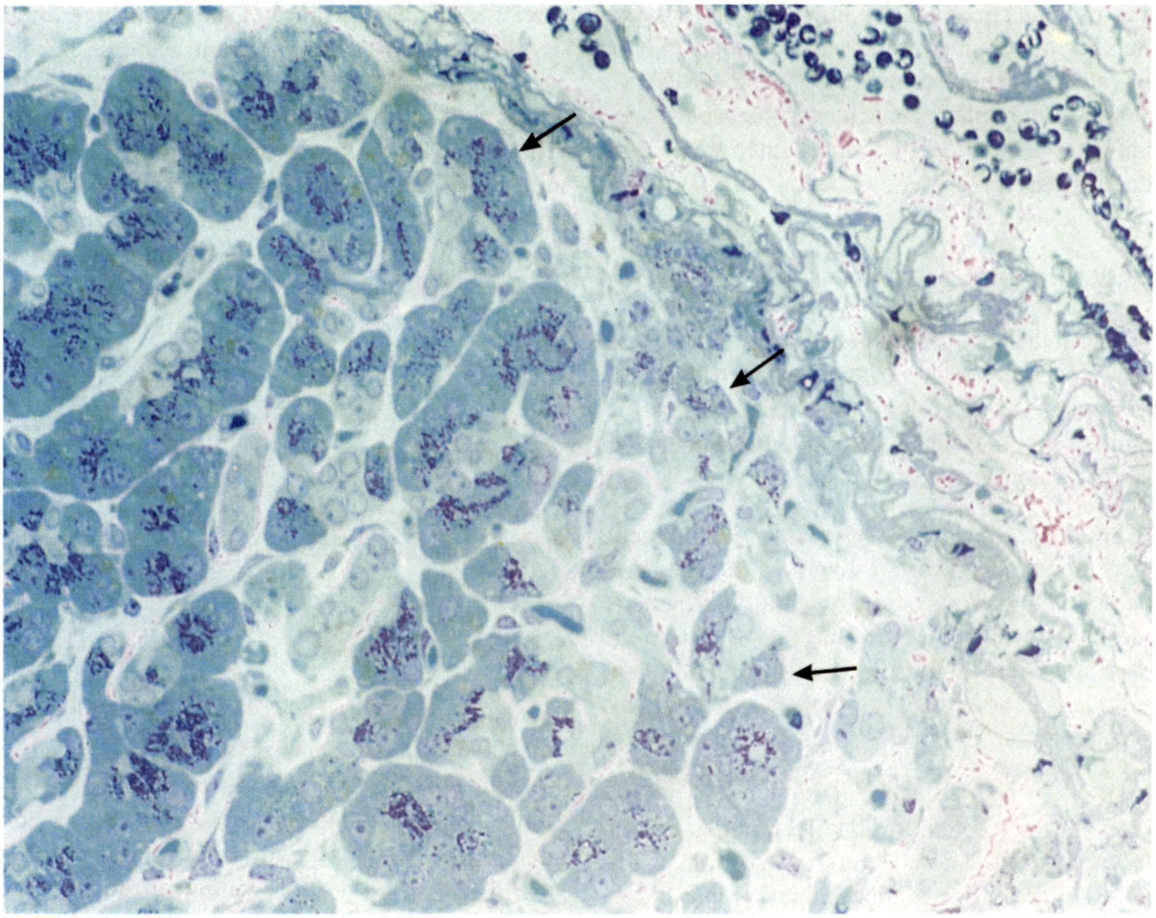

Fig. 30
Acute necrotizing pancreatitis. Edge of a fresh zone of necrosis (arrow). Deteriorating acinar cells. Fibrin deposits and haemorrhage in immediate vicinity of the parenchymal necrosis. Adjacent intact parenchymal zones exhibiting interstitial oedema.
Light micrograph
Semithin section
Stain: Basic fuchsin and methylene blue.
Magnification: 370 ×

necroses can spread in the omentum majus and in the fatty tissue of the renal capsules, especially on the left side. Colliquation necrosis can involve the complete glandular parenchyma. Sparse parenchymal residues can be maintained only in the periductal areas.

3.3.5.2 Microscopic Findings (Figs. 26–50)

In so-called oedematous pancreatitis an oedematous saturation of the acinar structure without alteration of the individual components can be recognized histologically. Only scattered fat necroses can be demonstrated.

In the haemorrhagic-necrotizing form of pancreatitis fat necroses initially dominate the histologic picture. They are developed within the organ, especially, however, in the outer zone. They are often interspersed with haemorrhages. in a time period of 12 hours to 2 days increasing parenchymal necroses arise, which can exhibit variably large haemorrhages (Schmitz-Moormann 1987).

Electron microscopically a large number of individual findings allow the reconstruction of the course of the initial reaction. Initial cytoplasmic alterations of the acinar epithelial cells can be found in allograft-pancreatitis, which is identical to genuine pancreatitis in its course and with reference to the histomorphological substrate. Vacuolization of the cells develops, arising from a pronounced dilatation of the cisterns of the endoplasmic reticulum and a reduction of the zymogen granula. Additionally a system consisting of secretory vacuoles with relatively uniform granular contents develops as in experimental pancreatitis induced by caerulin administration (Kern 1987). It can be observed that the zymogen granula dissolve in the vacuoles and their contrast-rich contents merge with the contents of the vacuoles. It is a point of discussion that probably owing to hypoxia a blockade in the endoplasmic reticulum occurs, preventing synthesis of the proenzymes. Due to the alterations in the intracytoplasmic transport systems the intermediate products arising during impaired synthesis are probably deposited in the vacuoles. It is conceivable that entrance of the zymogen granula into the vacuoles gives rise to intracytoplasmic activation of the proenzymes. The basal cell membrane can dissolve, probably elicited by intracellular enzyme activation. Zymogen granula enter the interstitial connective tissue by the membrane defect. Transmission and scanning electron microscopic findings show that individual granula in immediate vicinity of the affected cells initially remain intact in their outer form. The bordering membranes dissolve owing to the increasing enzyme activation taking place in the interstitium, the contents of the granula thus being able to be released into the intercellular fluid.

Components of the cytoplasm such as fragments of the endoplasmic reticulum and deteriorating mitochondria lie exposed in the interstitial connective tissue. In the area of the dissolving acinar cells fibrin deposits develop. The collagen fibres break up, forming short fragments. Necrosis extends to the capillary walls. Gaps are found in the endothelium, by which the erythrocytes can enter adjacent necrotic parts of the connective tissue. In vicinity of the endothelial defects thrombocyte aggregates with fibrin deposits form. In scanning electron microscopy a mixture of zymogen granula, cytoplasmic fragments of the acinar cells, deteriorating erythrocytes and fibrin deposits can be demonstrated in the zone of necrosis.

Fig. 31
Early intracytoplasmic alterations in an acinar epithelial cell after pancreatic transplantation. A system consisting of secretory vacuoles develops, to which the zymogen granula line up against. Regular granular contents of the vacuoles. Scattered zymogen granula migrate to the vacuolar lumen (arrow).
Transmission electron micrograph
Magnification: 8500 ×

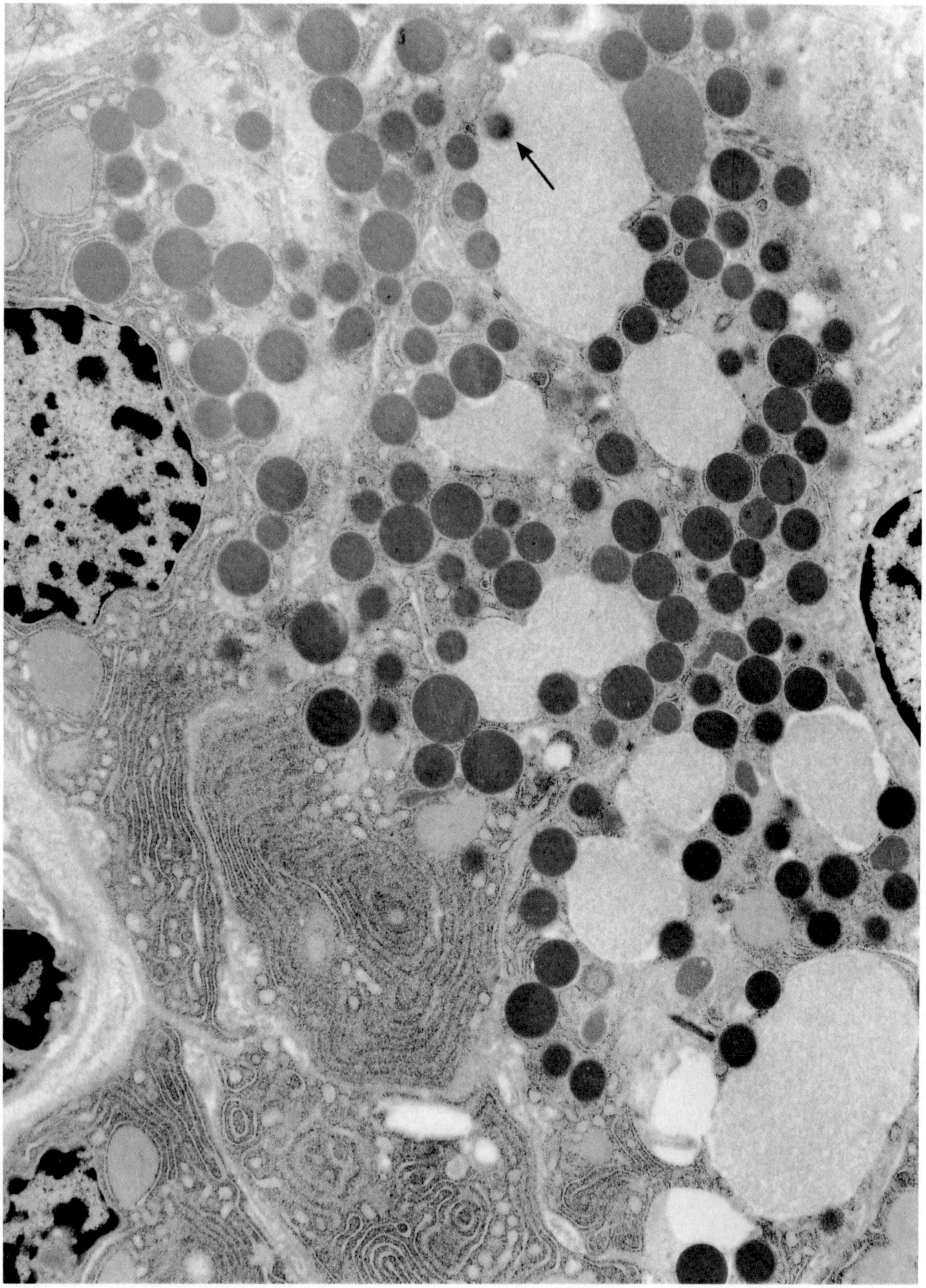

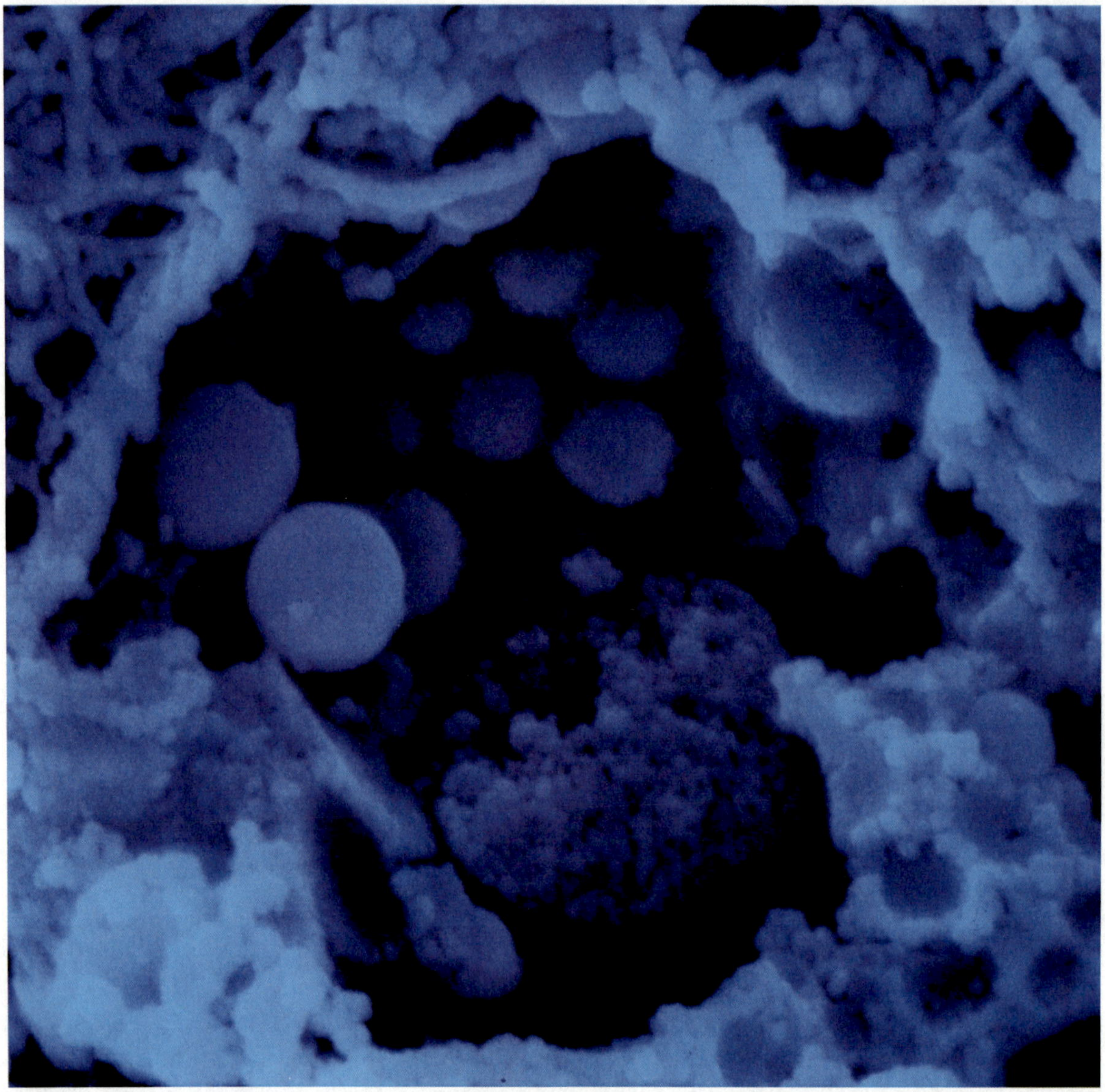

Fig. 32
Secretory vacuole in the cytoplasm of an acinar epithelial cell after pancreatic transplantation. The zymogen granula lined up against the vacuolar membrane indent the membrane. 2 granula have migrated to the lumina of the vacuoles. Behind it granular contents of the vacuole.
Scanning electron micrograph
Magnification: 11300 ×

Fig. 33
Alteration of the acinar cells in acute necrotizing pancreatitis. In intact parenchymal zones outside of the necroses irregular oedematous dispersion of the acinar cells. Variable degree of vesicular cisterns of the endoplasmic reticulum. Irregular distribution of the zymogen granula in the acinar cells. Variable density of the karyoplasm in the cellular nuclei. Marked interstitial oedema with loosening of the fibre structures. ▷
Transmission electron micrograph
Magnification: 6500 ×

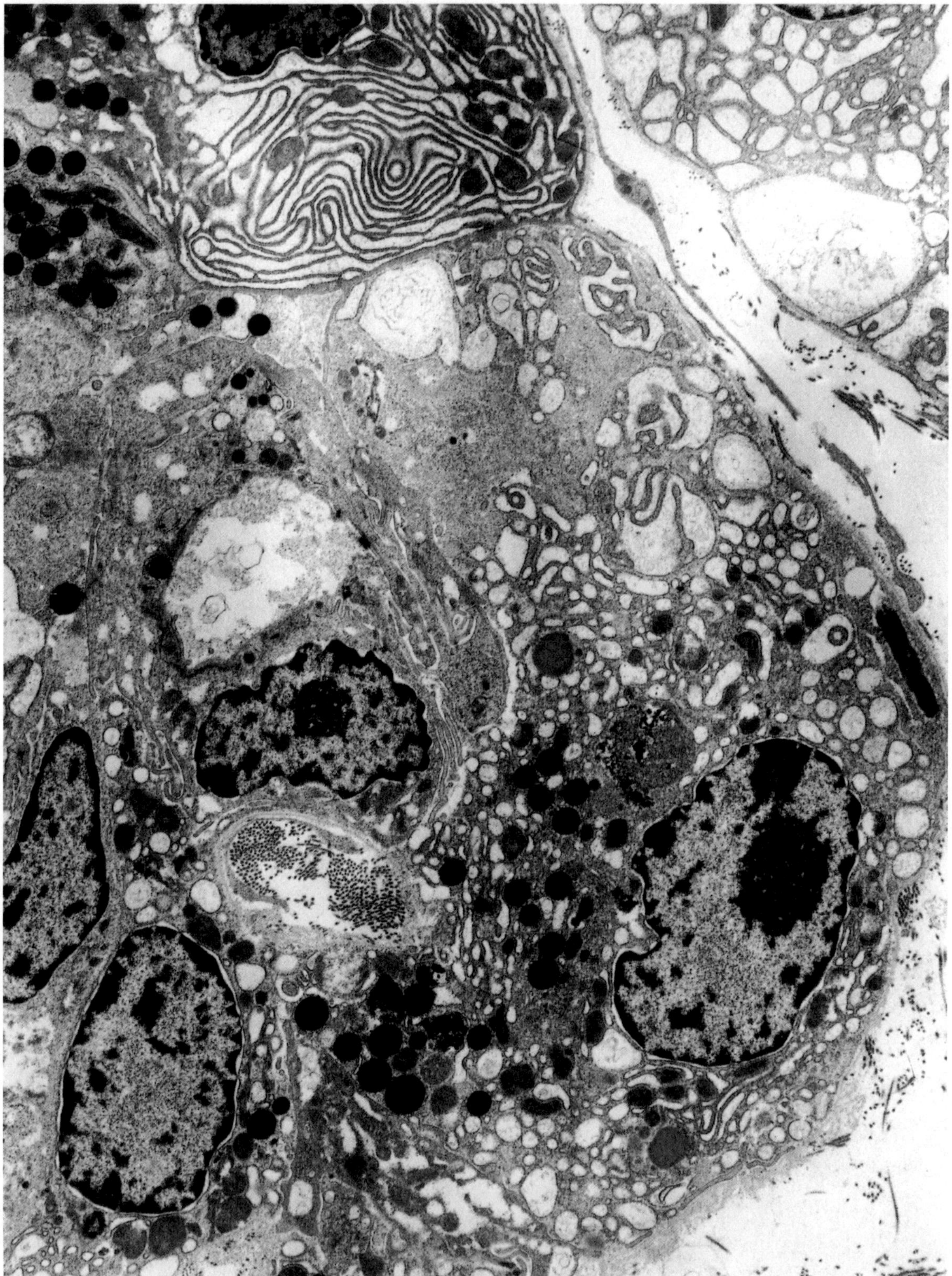

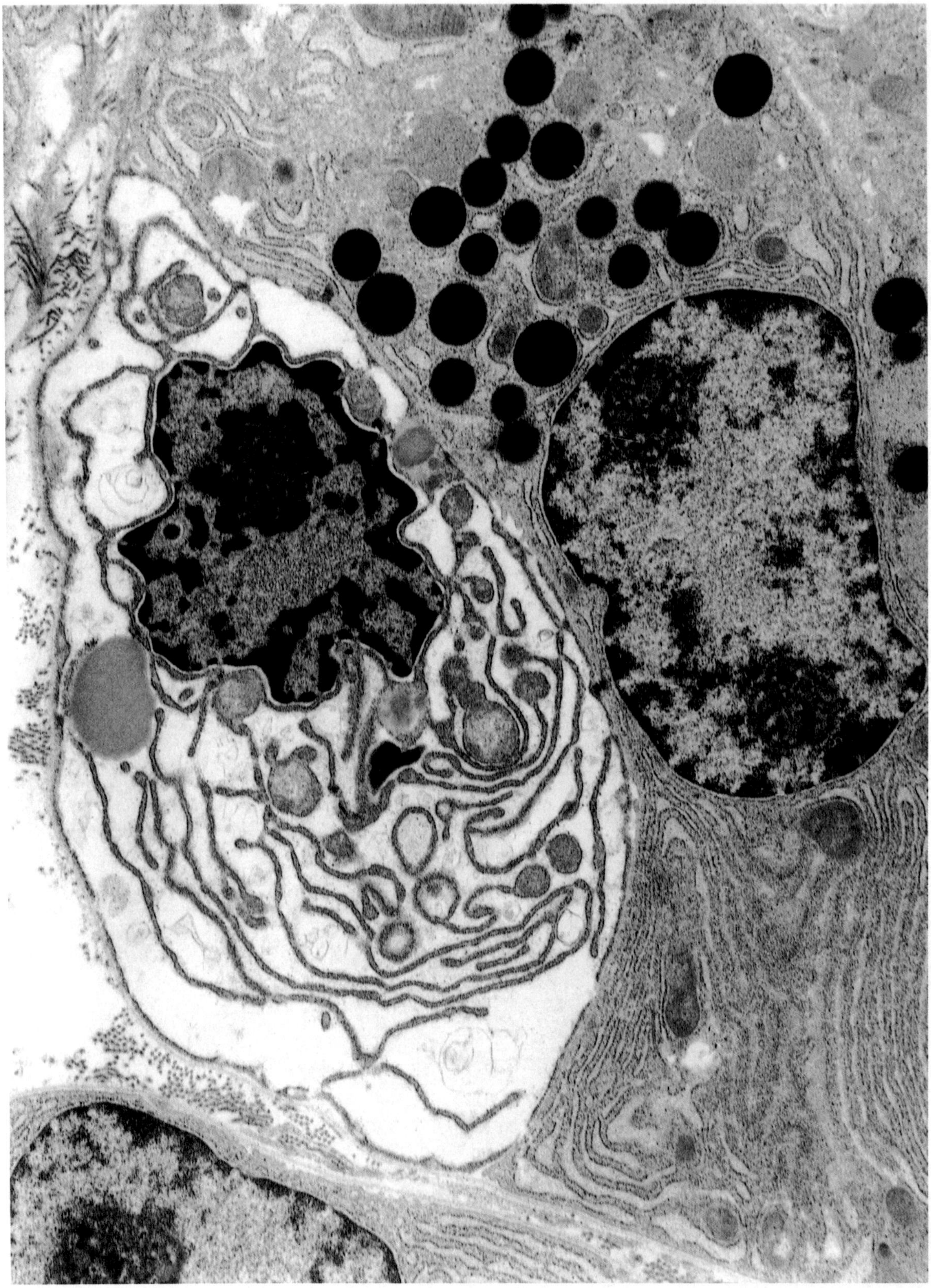

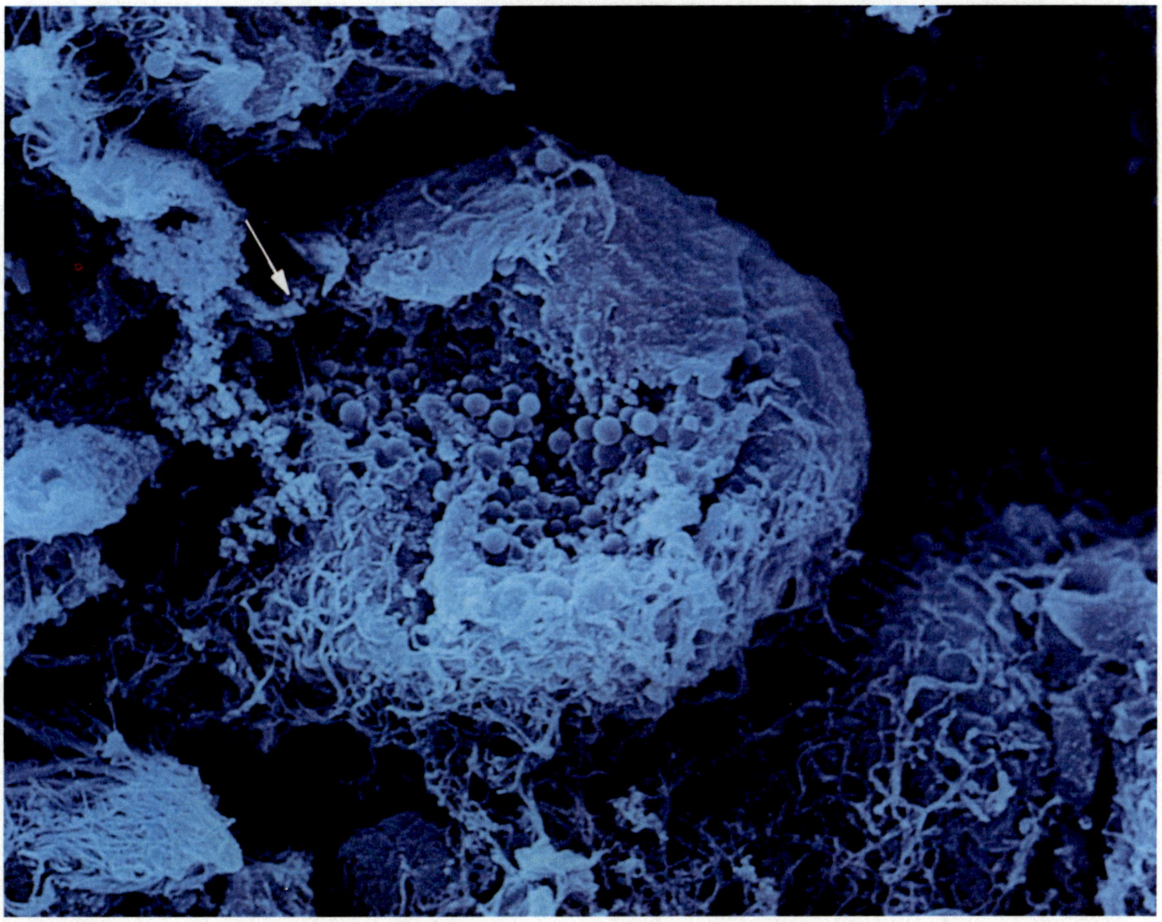

◁ Fig. 34
Marked interstitial oedema of an acinar cell in the vicinity of a recent pancreatic necrosis. Prominent distension of the cisterns of the endoplasmic reticulum. Complete extinction of secretory action. Condensation of the karyoplasm in the cellular nucleus. Formation of deep indentations in the cellular nucleus and nuclear shrinkage. Mitochondria between parts of the endoplasmic reticulum.
Transmission electron micrograph
Magnification: 13000 ×

Fig. 35
Edge of fresh necrosis of the pancreatic parenchyma. Broad opening in the cell membrane (arrow). Liberation of zymogen granula into the oedematous, loosened interstitium.
Scanning electron micrograph
Magnification: 4800 ×

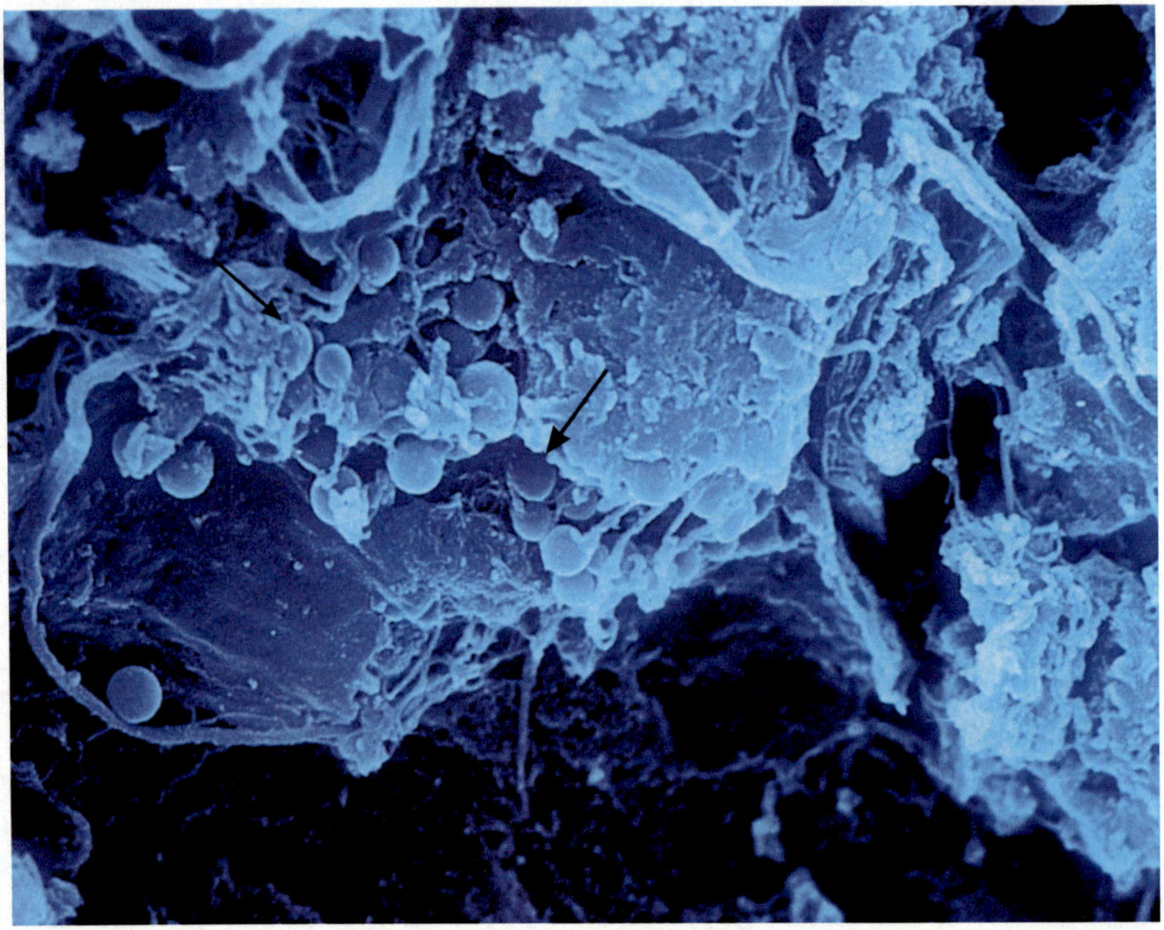

Fig. 36
Liberation of zymogen granula into the interstitium of the marginal zone of a fresh parenchymal necrosis. The zymogen granula reach the interstitium via openings in the cell membrane in the basolateral and basal cellular zones (arrows). Marked oedematous loosening of the interstitial connective tissue structure. Adjacent irregularly circumscribed granular detritus material and fibrin deposits.
Scanning electron micrograph
Magnification: 7500 ×

Fig. 37
Edge of a fresh pancreatic necrosis with release of zymogen ▷ granula into the interstitium (arrows) from decomposing acinar cells. Adjacent to the necrotic epithelial cells variably broad, lamellar fibrin deposits. In the acinar cells vesicular transgression of the mitochondria and dilatation of the cisterns of the endoplasmic reticulum. Irregular distension of the intercellular spaces.
Transmission electron micrograph
Magnification: 7000 ×

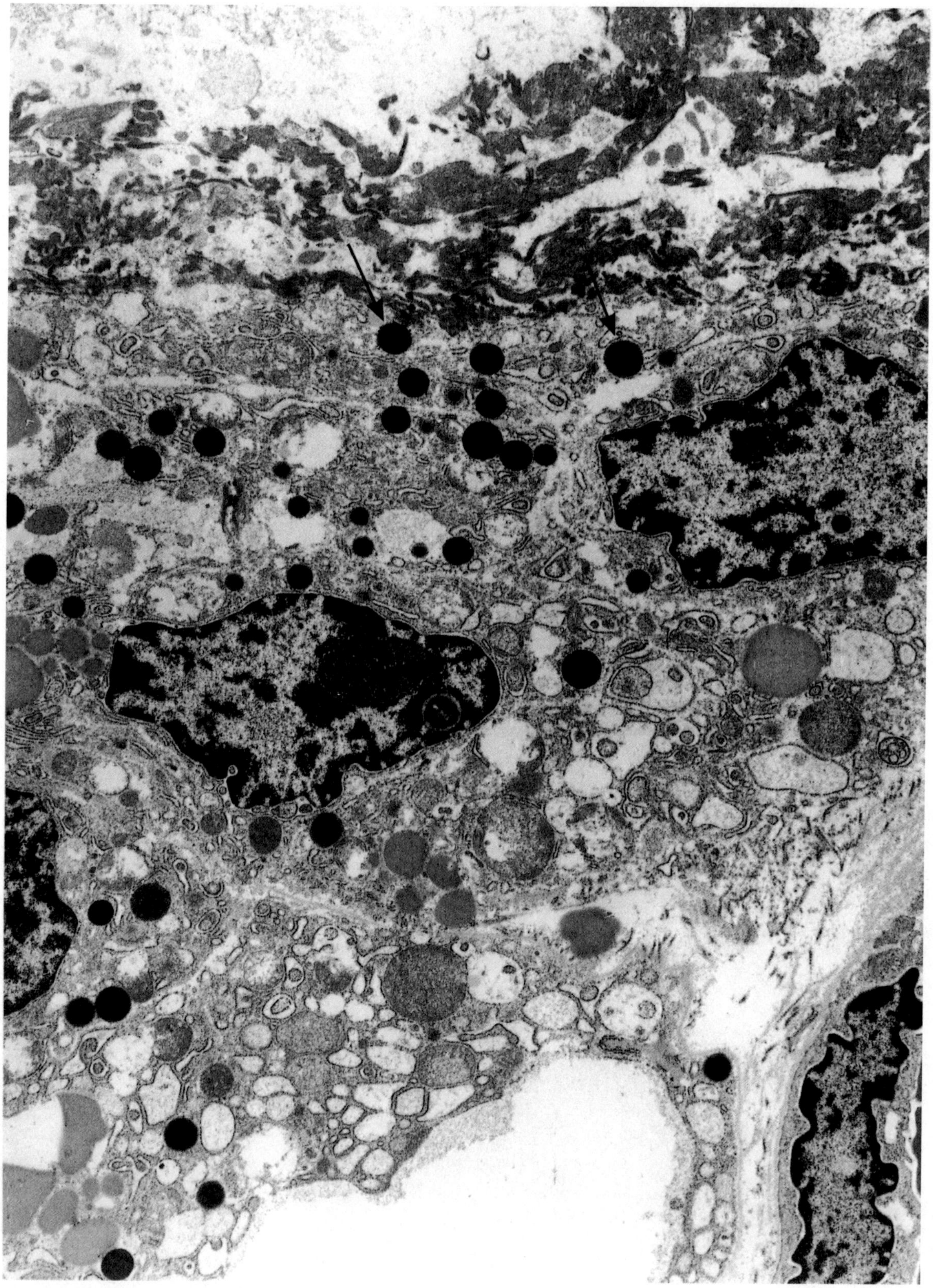

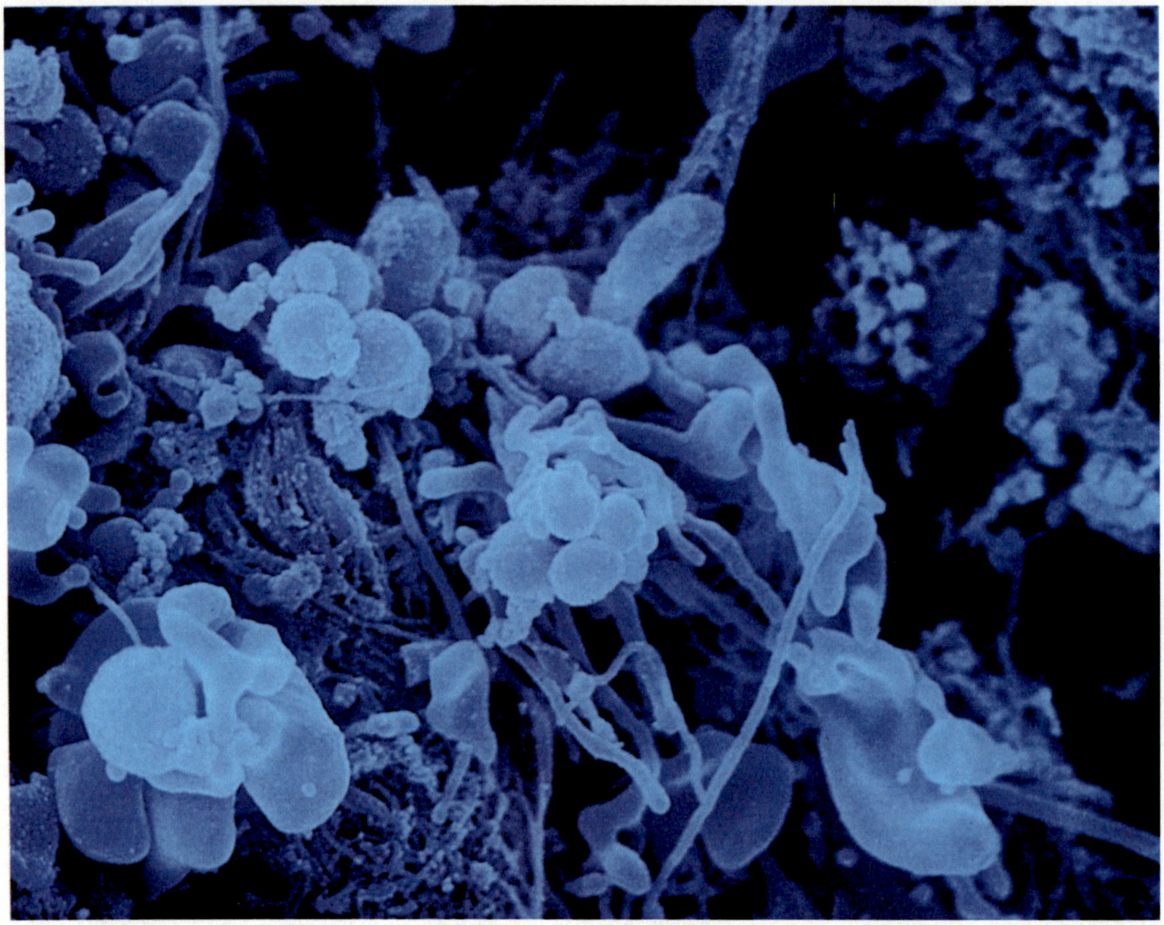

Fig. 58
Marginal zone of a fresh parenchymal necrosis. Release of intracytoplasmic structures into the interstitium. Aside from lamella of the endoplasmic reticulum and variably large mitochondria deteriorating zymogen granula. Adjacent irregular fibrin deposits and granular detritus material.
Scanning electron micrograph
Magnification: 7400 ×

Fig. 59
Extension of necrosis to a capillary wall. Formation of variably wide gaps in the endothelial lining (arrow). Aggregation of thrombocytes in vicinity of the endothelial defect. Spillage of erythrocytes into the interstitial, oedematous, loosened connective tissue (dark complexes at the right of the picture). ▷
Transmission electron micrograph
Magnification: 5100 ×

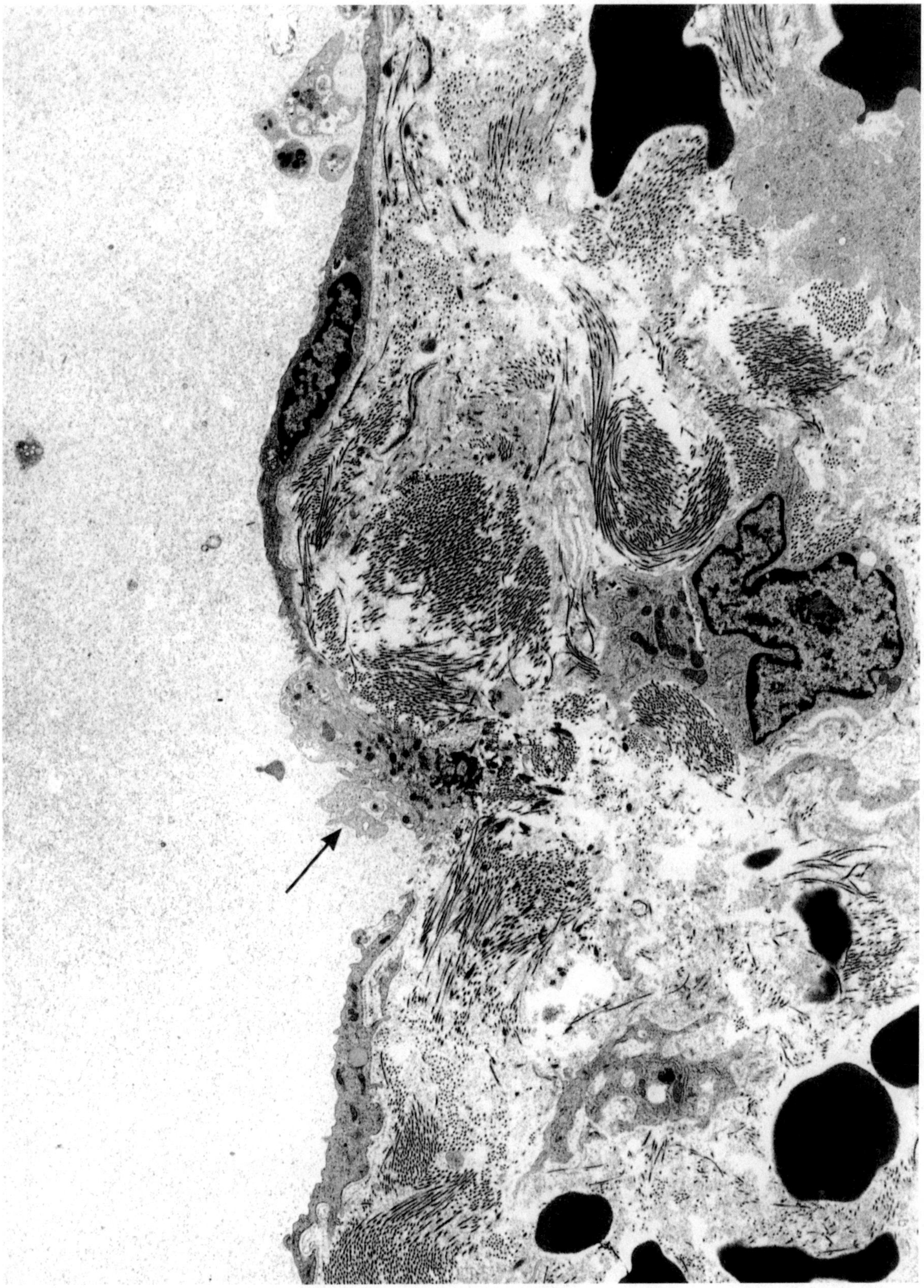

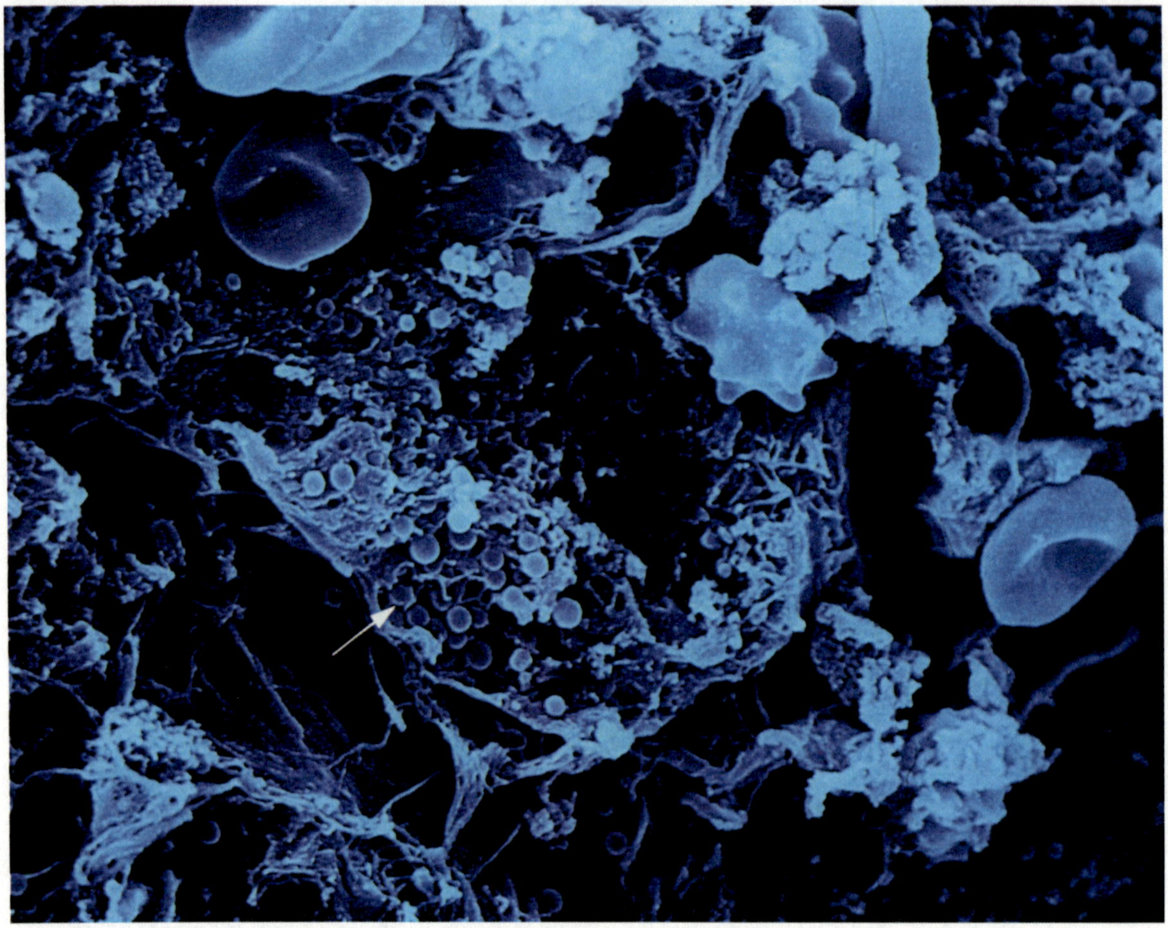

Fig. 40
Edge of a fresh parenchymal necrosis with haemorrhage. Beside decomposing acinar cells (arrows) variably broad, thready fibrin deposits. Inbetween variably large complexes consisting of cellular detritus. Embedded in the cell detritus aggregates of erythrocytes. Formation of crenocytes. Adjacent pronounced distension of the intercellular spaces in neighboring areas of the acinar system.
Scanning electron micrograph
Magnification: 5700 ×

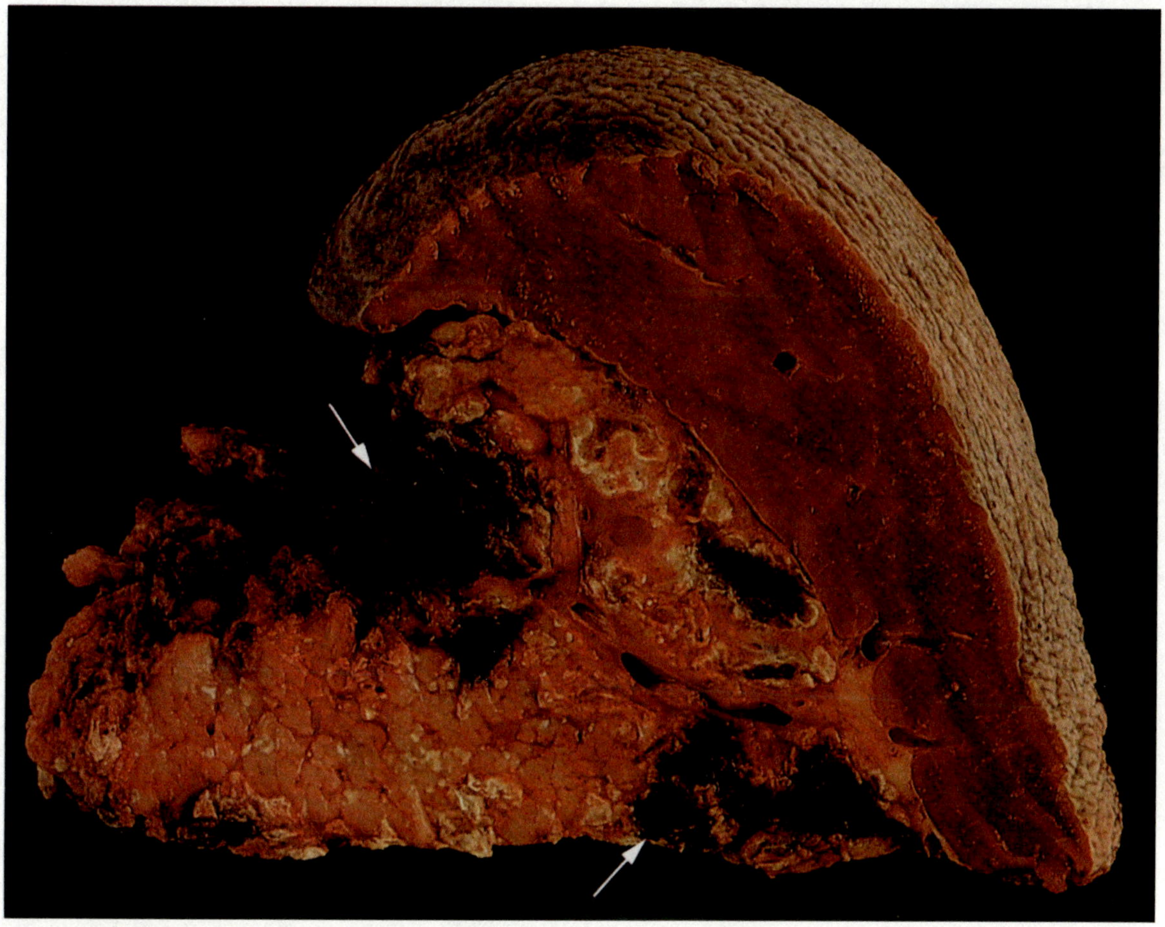

Fig. 41
Advanced haemorrhagic necrotizing pancreatitis in the pancreatic tail. Surgical specimen after left lateral pancreatic resection. Irregularly limited confluating necroses, darkly discolored owing to haemorrhage, which extends into the fatty tissue of the splenic hilum (arrows).

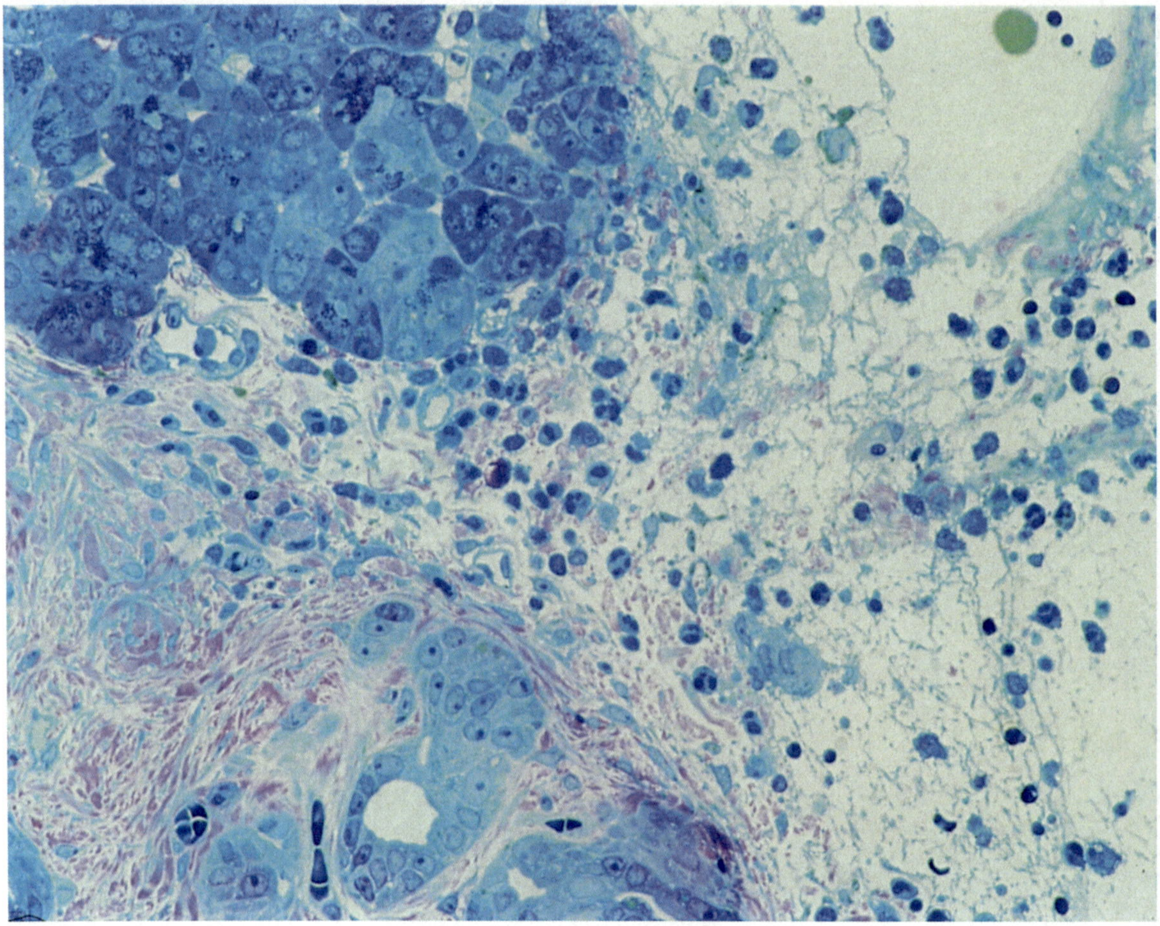

Fig. 42
Beginning organization of pancreatic necrosis. Migration of granulocytes and macrophages to the zone of necrosis. Within the necroses netlike, finely filamentous fibrin structure.
Semithin section
Stain: Basic fuchsin and methylene blue
Magnification: 390 ×

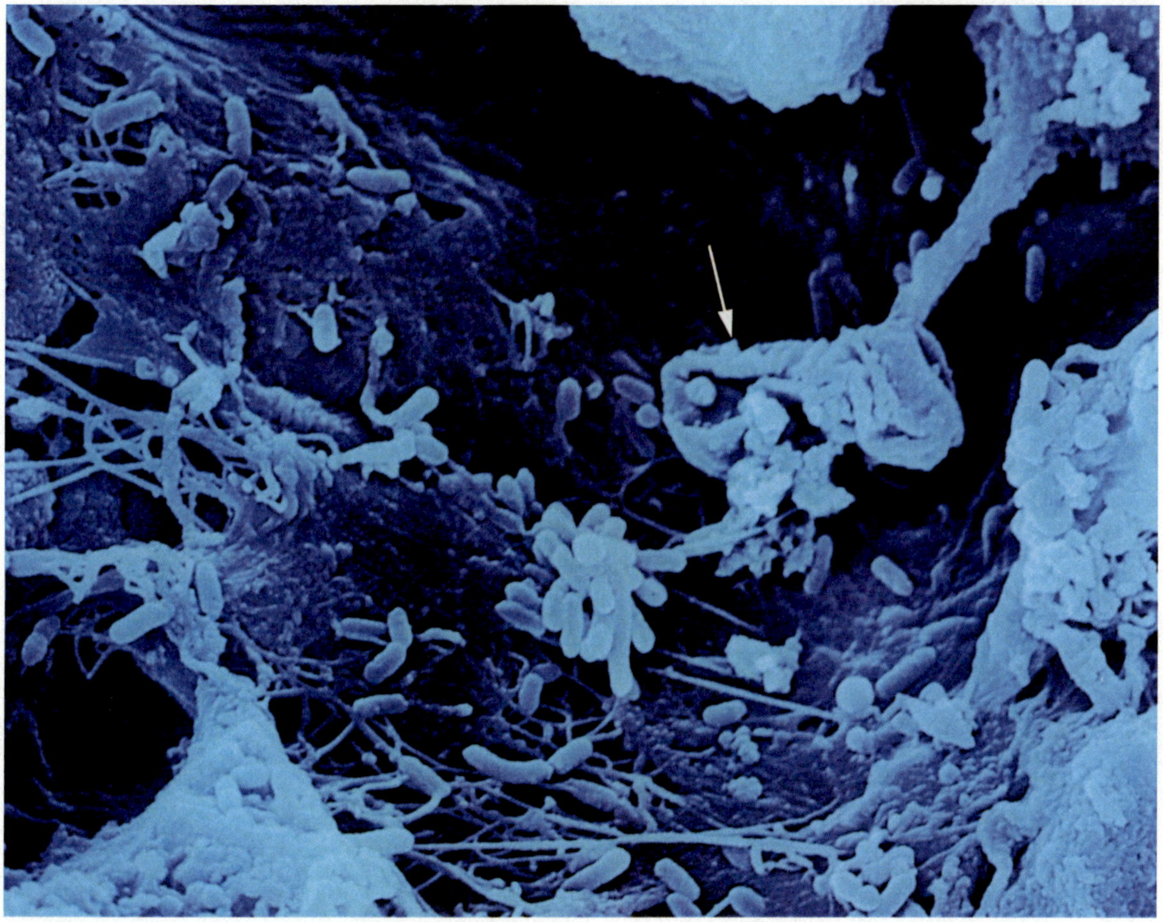

Fig. 43
Bacterial colonization of pancreatic necrosis. At the edge of the necrosis variably large complexes of rod-shaped bacteria. The bacteria approach a protrusion of a macrophage (arrow) with a trunk-like structure at the tip of the protrusions for phagocytosis of the bacteria. Adjacent finely filamentous fibrin deposits in the marginal zone of the necrosis.
Scanning electron micrograph
Magnification: 6300 ×

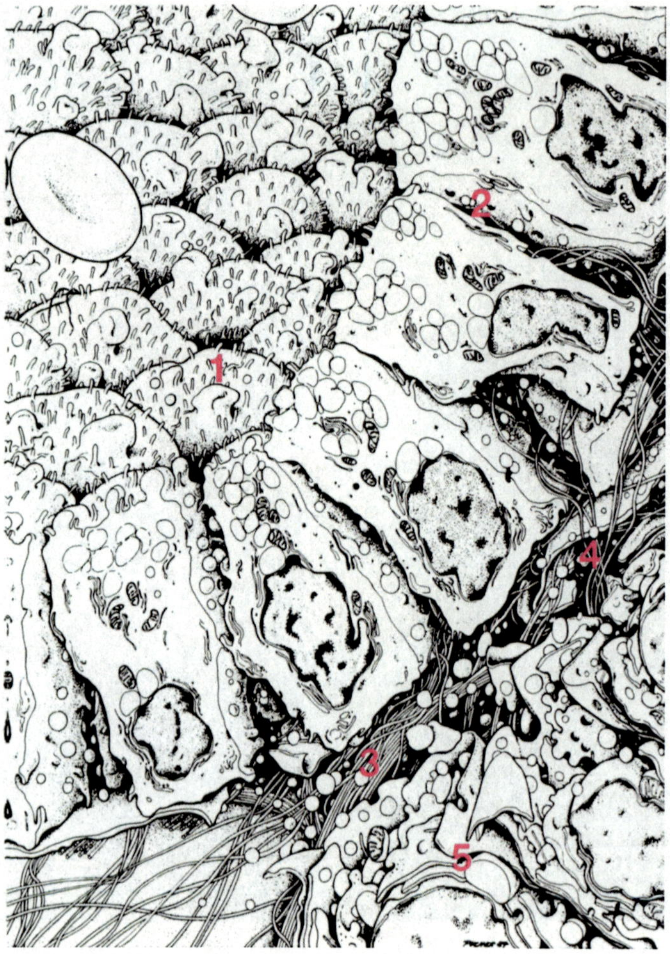

Fig. 44
Alterations of the ductal system surrounding pancreatic necroses. Partial loss of the microvilli structure. Gross distensions of the cell surface as an indication of intracellular oedema. Distension of the intercellular spaces. Open connection of the ductal lumen with the interstitium. Release of zymogen granula from deteriorating acinar cells into the periductal connective tissue matrix loosened by oedema.

1. Alteration of the microvilli structure at the epithelial surface with formation of gross distensions.
2. Distension of the intercellular space and dissolution of the intercellular contact zones.
3. Zymogen granula released into the interstitium.
4. Oedema in the interstitium with loosening of the fibre structure.
5. Deteriorating acinar cells.

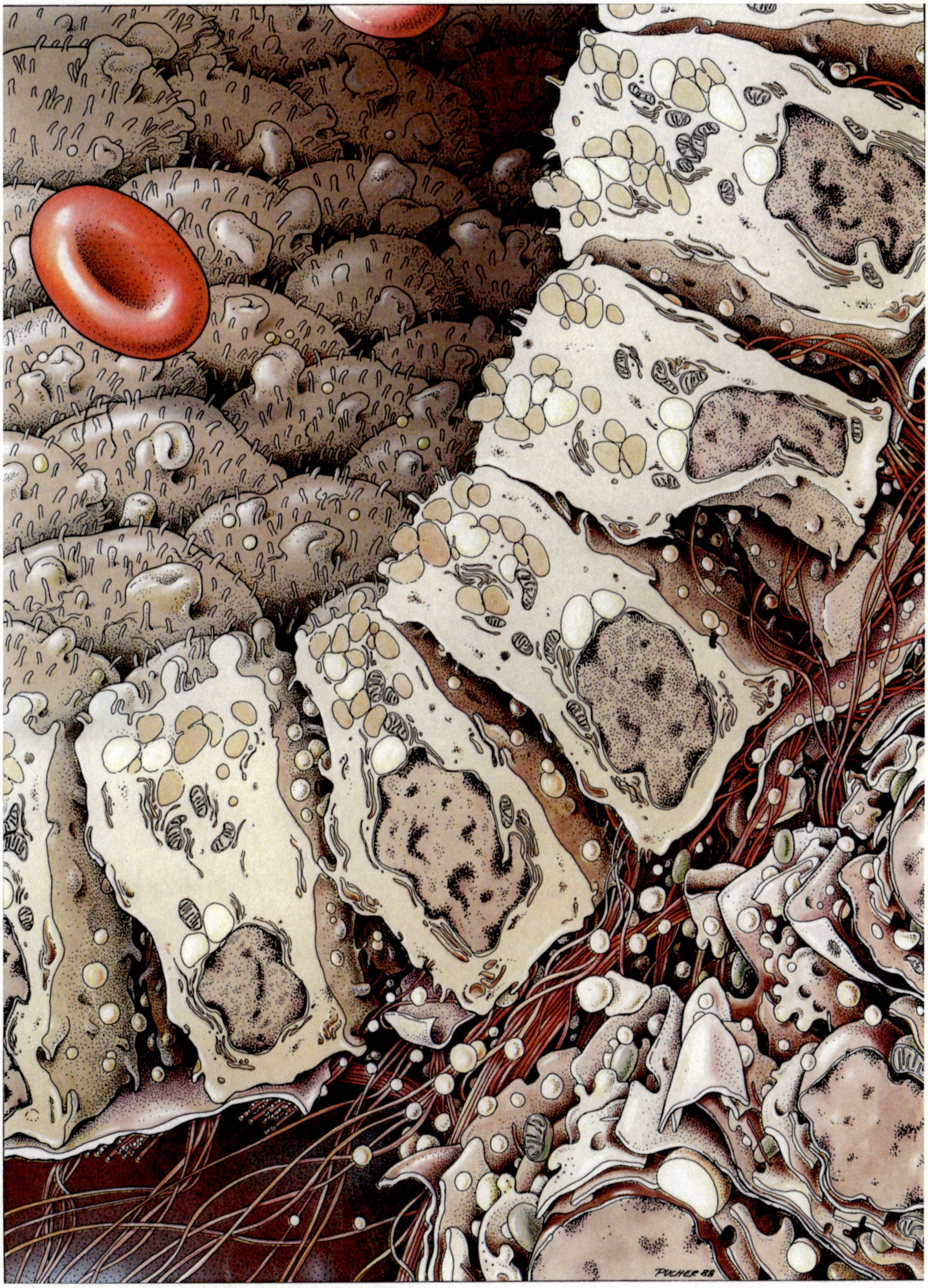
PUCHER 88

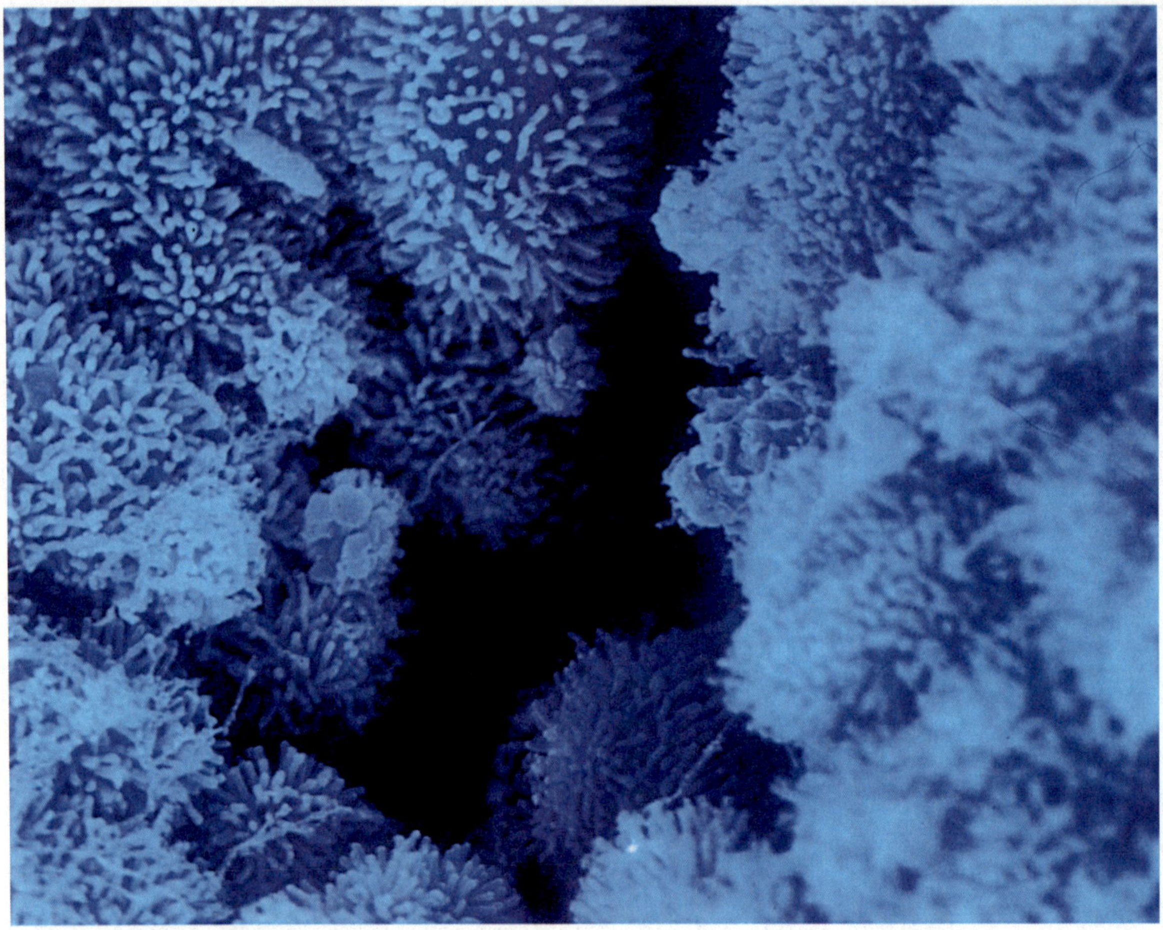

Fig. 45
Alterations of the ductal epithelium. Dissolution of the intercellular contact zones with formation of wide intercellular spaces. Irregular microvilli structure at the surface of the individual epithelial cells. Above the epithelium scattered mucous threads and complexes composed of zymogen granula.
Scanning electron micrograph
Magnification: 7900 ×

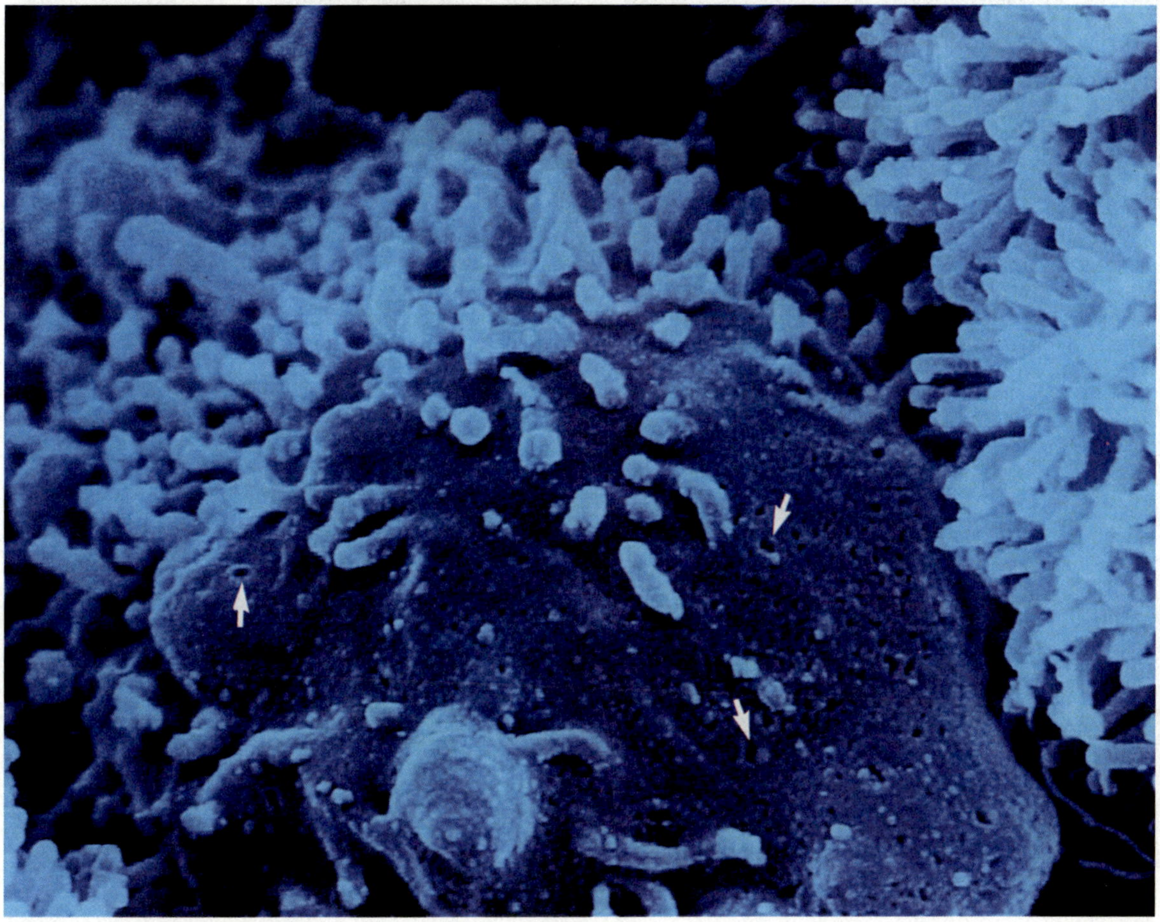

Fig. 46
Alterations of the ductal epithelium surrounding a pancreatic necrosis. Partial loss of the microvilli structure at the surface of the ductal epithelial cells. Punched out appearing defects in the cell membrane (arrows) as an indication of beginning cell deterioration. Adjacent dissolution of intercellular contacts with formation of wide intercellular spaces.
Scanning electron micrograph
Magnification: 16500 ×

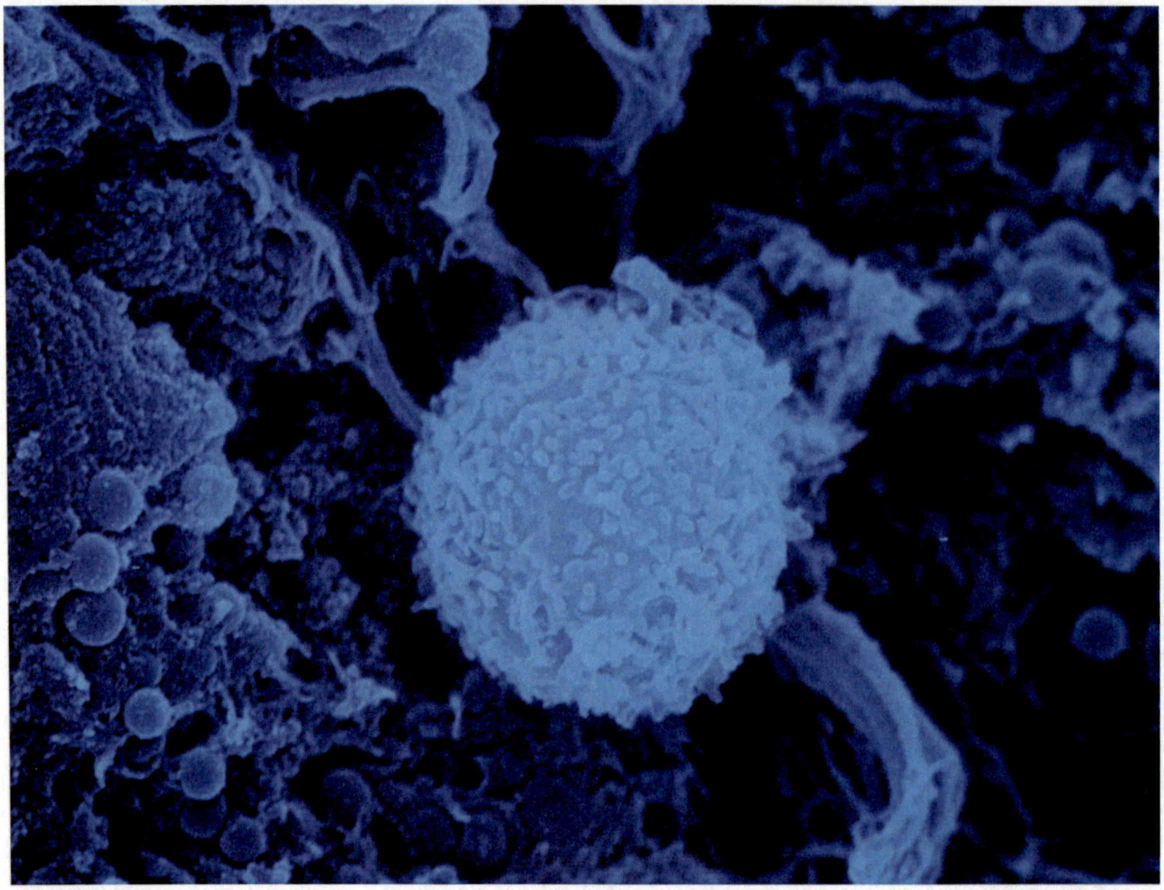

Fig. 47

Beginning organization of pancreatic necrosis. Granulocytes and macrophages migrate to zones of necrosis. At the macrophage surface microvilli and microplicae. The macrophages approach fibrin deposits and the rest of the dissolving acinar epithelial cells and ingest the substances by phagocytosis.

Scanning electron micrograph
Magnification: 7600 ×

Fig. 48

Organization of pancreatic necrosis. In vicinity of the reaction loose infiltrates consisting of lymphocytes, scattered granulocytes and many macrophages. Activation of fibroblasts with production of new fibres. Variably broad fascicles of collagen fibres between the cells. ▷

Transmission electron micrograph
Magnification: 5400 ×

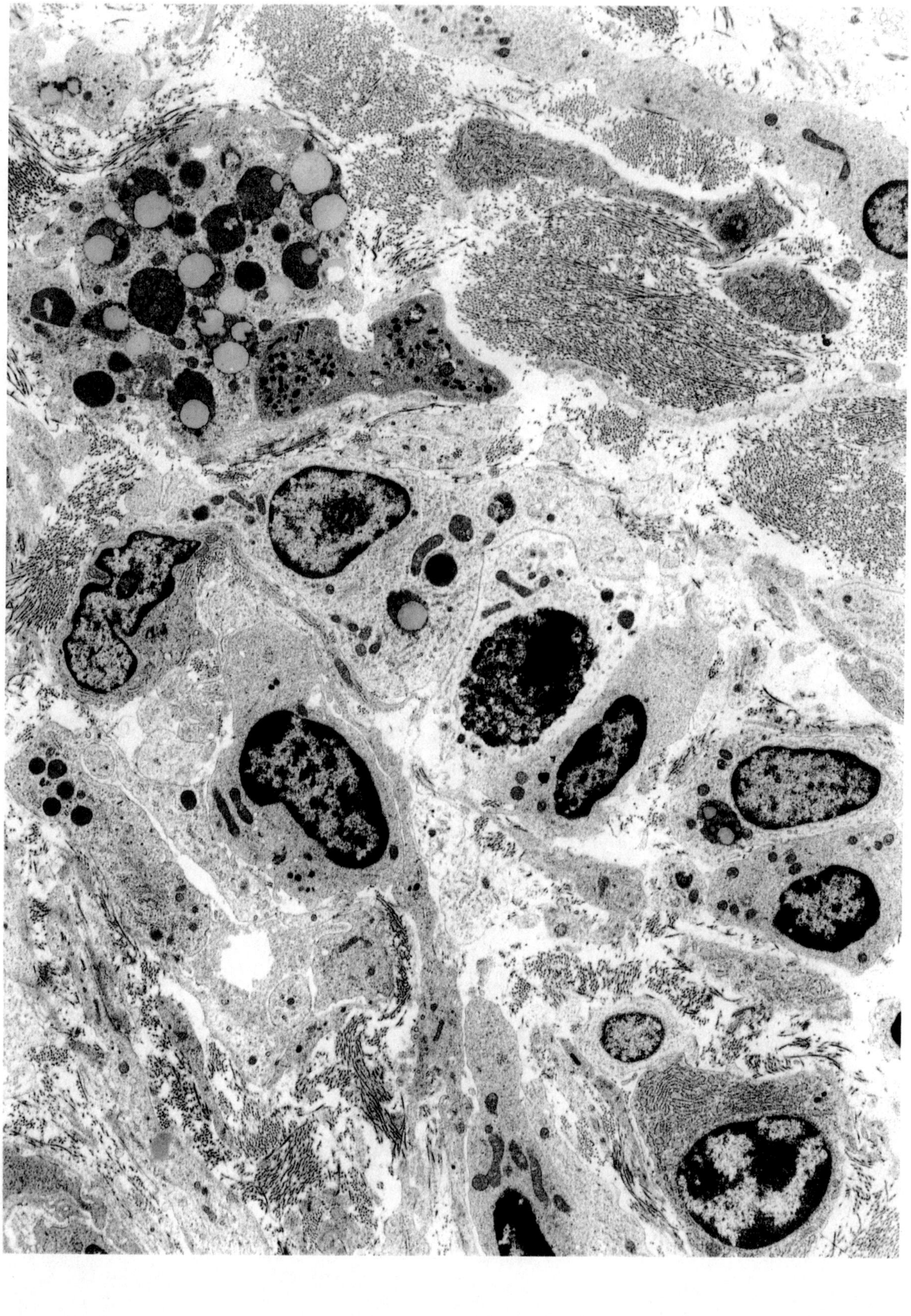

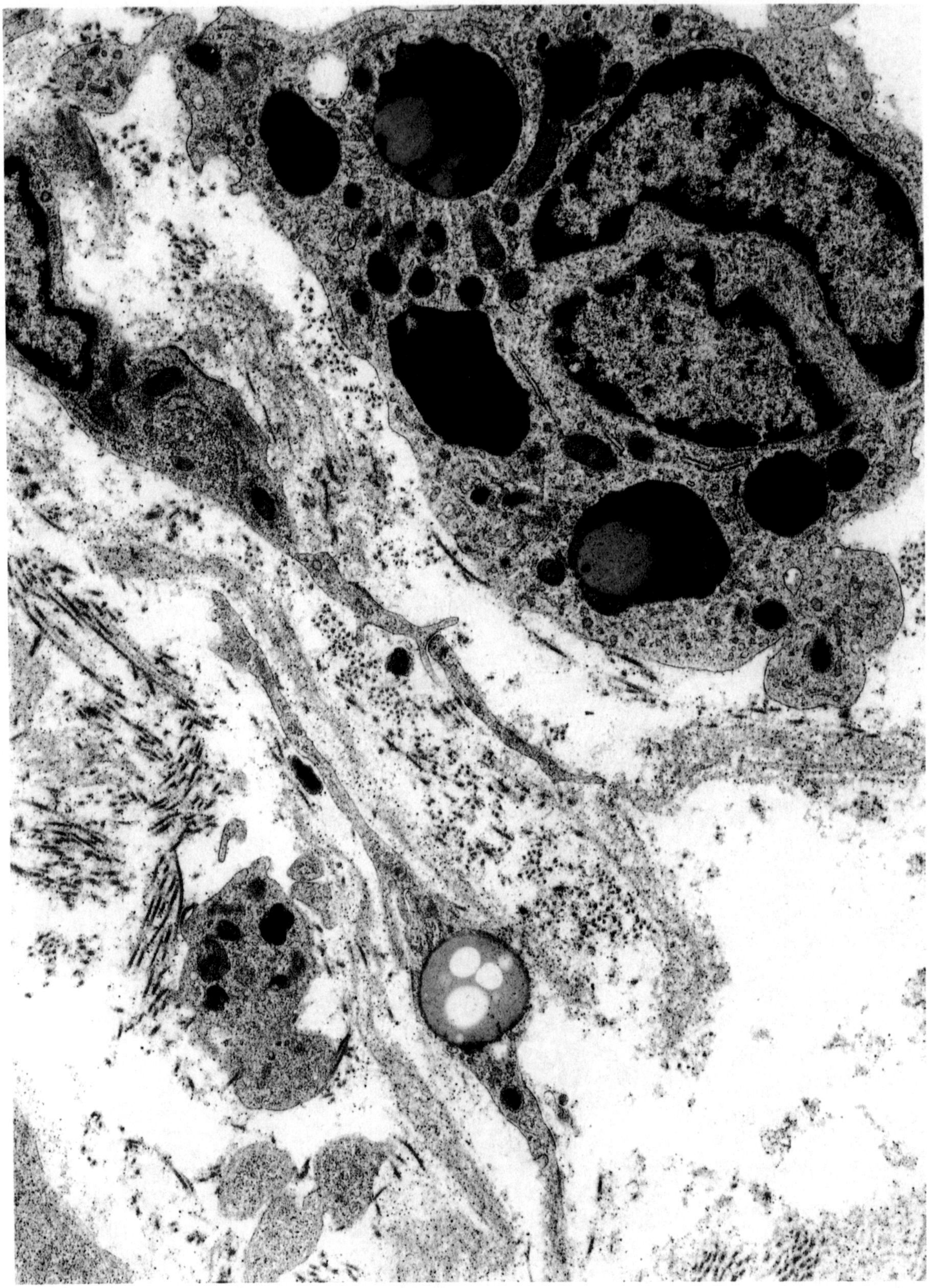

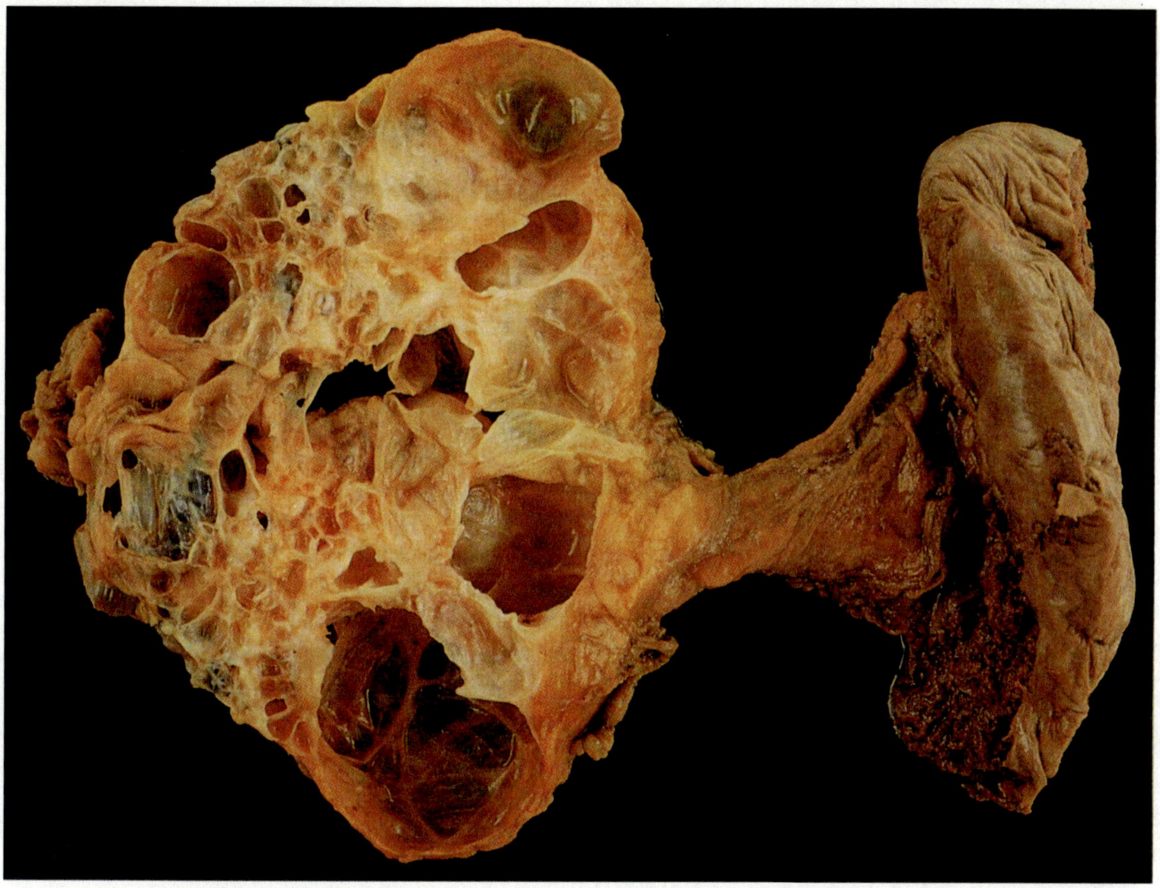

◁ Fig. 49
Macrophages at the marginal zone of a pancreatic necrosis in organization. Large macrophages containing variably large phagolysosomes. Eccentrically located, deeply indented cellular nucleus. Adjacent active fibroblasts exhibiting formation of new fibres.
Transmission electron micrograph
Magnification: 13300 ×

Fig. 50
Complete pseudocystic transformation of the pancreatic head following acute pancreatic necrosis. Surgical specimen. In vicinity of the pancreatic head broad cavities with smooth inner surfaces limited by richly fibrous connective tissue. Marked fibrosis in the area of the pancreatic tail.

Granulocytes enter the necrosis from the vascular lumina. Macrophages characterized by a differentiated system of microvilli at the cell surface come to lie alongside of cellular fragments and deteriorating erythrocytes and pass them via phagocytosis into the cytoplasm.

The components enveloped by the cytoplasmic phagolysosomes exhibit variable degrees of intracellular lytic degradation. In vicinity of the necroses marked alterations of the ductal epithelium can be found. Distension of the intercellular spaces develops from the epithelial surface to the basal lamella, so that constituents of the pancreatic secretions from the lumen can reach the periductal connective tissue zone.

As an expression of epithelial cell swelling the microvilli become thick protrusions. In variably wide areas the microvilli structure can flatten out completely. In the cell membrane punched out appearing membrane defects measuring up to 0.05 μm in diameter arise in these zones. Degenerative alterations with vacuolar distension of the endoplasmic reticulum in variable distribution can be observed.

In 2–5% of the cases (Schmitz-Moormann 1987) secondary bacterial colonization of the parenchymal necroses with liquification of tissue induced by the bacteria and granulocytic marginal reaction can be demonstrated. The bacteria are arranged in variably large groups between the constituents of the necroses and threads of fibrin. The bacteria can be ingested by granulocytes as well as macrophages by means of phagocytosis. The macrophages initially approach the cytoplasmic extensions of the microorganisms. At the beginning of phagocytosis a mouth-shaped trough develops in the cell membrane so that a trunk-like structure arises at the cell surface.

The morphologic substrate of the late stage in the course of acute pancreatitis is characterized by the organization of necroses and development of fibrosis, which can especially spread out in peripancreatic areas forming a mantle-shaped, scarred zone. Variably large scarred regions develop, in which remains of the acinar structure and the duct system are enclosed. In larger areas the islets often remain intact, even when complete necrosis of the acinar system has occurred. In this healing phase pseudocysts and abscesses owing to bacterial superinfections of the necroses are the most important local complications (Schmitz-Moormann 1987). Infection of the peripancreatic tissue and the peripancreatic exudate are held responsible for abscess formation.

Liquification of the necroses in the larger zone of necrosis sealed off by granulation and scarred tissue are the basis allowing the development of pseudocysts. These can be demonstrated with visual aids during the post-acute stage of acute pancreatitis in up to 50% of the cases (Dürr 1979). In the further course part of the pseudocysts are completely transformed into scars. If a connection exists between the pseudocysts and the ductal system they receive enzyme-rich fluid. In correspondence with the location of necrosis pseudocysts arising in acute pancreatitis are located mainly in the parapancreatic tissue and are rare in central parts of the pancreatic parenchyma.

3.3.6 Therapy of Acute Pancreatitis

As the course of the disease and the prognosis cannot be assessed reliably at the onset of acute pancreatitis careful and regular controls are focus of therapy, at least in the first week of the disease. Patients with imminent and manifest severe cases must be under continuous observation in the intensive care unit. The circulatory parameters blood pressure and pulse rate, palpation and auscultation of the abdomen, supervision of fluid intake and output, central venous pressure and laboratory values of haemoglobin and or haematocrit, the number of leucocytes, amylase levels in the serum and urine and/or lipase in the serum, serum calcium, blood glucose daily profile, serum potassium, urea, creatinine in the serum, arterial pO_2-pressure, acid-base-balance and sonography of the upper abdomen, the latter in 1–3 day intervals, are especially suitable for patient monitoring. Regular clinical examinations offer important clues anticipating imminent deterioration which often precede laboratory findings (Bohnsack et al. 1983).

3.3.6.1 Conservative Therapy

First and foremost aims of therapy are symptomatical supportive measures for treatment and prophylaxis of clinical sequels of the severe inflammatory condition in the upper abdomen. Causal therapy is impossible, especially because in severe cases essential pathogenetic mechanisms have already taken their course before therapy is begun with. It primarily applies to eliminate hypovolemic shock by administration of sufficient fluids, electrolytes, albumin and blood transfusions in case of severe haemorrhaging, as well as elimination of pain, as ensuing vasodilation intensifies hypovolemic shock. Careful attention must further be paid to the development of respiratory failure and in case of falling arterial oxygen pressure administration of oxygen or in serious cases assisted respiration must be begun with in time (see diagram below). Further aims in therapy are correction of an acute diabetic metabolic situation with insulin or of hypalbuminemia, hypocalcemia or replacement of electrolytes as the case may be. It is important to check for possibly developing local complications such as abscess formation with sepsis, development of large pseudocysts with haemorrhage or bronchopneumonia. Measures to suppress secretory activity and so-called "putting the pancreas to rest" have proved disappointing (see below).

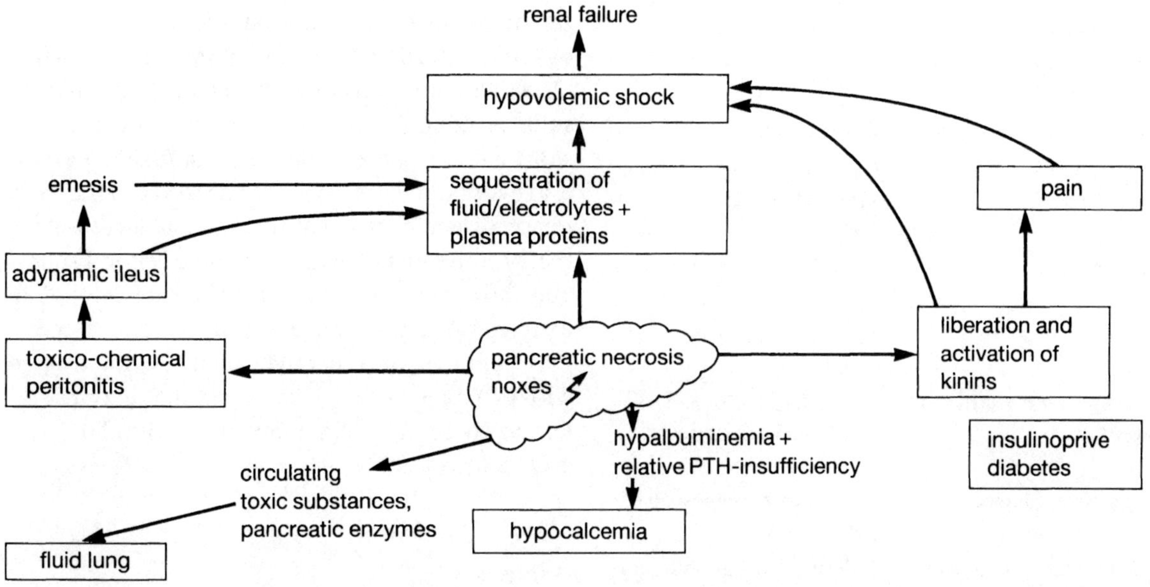

Pathophysiology of acute pancreatitis as the approach to therapy

Table 7 Standard basic treatment in acute pancreatitis

Hospital Referral/Surveillance
Starvation diet, if necessary gastric tube
Parenteral electrolyte-sugar-amino acid-mixture (2.5–3 l/24 h
Additionally spasmoanalgesics, morphine derivatives
Antibiotics (ampicillin, mezlocillin, cephalosporines) in severe alcoholic and in all non-alcoholic types
Not obligatory: synthetic salmon-calcitonin 60 μg = 300MRC-U/24 h for adjuvant stabilisation

Table 8 Supplementary program in the treatment of acute pancreatitis

Symptom	Measures
Shock	Administration of liquids (if necessary human albumin) according to central venous pressure
Hb-HK-drop	Full blood
Fever, Sepsis	Antibiotics (ampicillin, mezlocillin, cephalosporines, etc.)
Renal failure	Haemodialysis (if necessary in the early phase of severe cases, peritoneal dialysis)
Respiratory failure (pO_2-drop higher than 15 mm Hg or pO_2 lower than 60 mm Hg)	Assisted Respiration (Desired pO_2 80–120 mm Hg)
Encephalopathie	O_2-Application
Hypocalcemia	Calcium gluconate i. v., possibly additional human albumin
Hypokalemia	Potassium replenishment i. v.
Hyperglycemia	Regular insulin in small doses
In severe cases: gastric pH lower than 4	Cimetidine additionally to calcitonin i. v. for stress ulcer prophylaxis
Progressive jaundice	ERC, possibly endoscopic papillotomy
In foudroyant progression	Indication for early surgery
In local delayed complications	If necessary surgical intervention

Basic program (Table 7) and supplementary program (Table 8)

In the early painful stage abstinence from food is recommended in all cases. The gastric tube should only be administered as long as severe upper abdominal symptoms with emesis and signs of subileus are present. In quick improvement of the clinical condition probatory removal of the gastric tube can be performed and the patient can be given unsweetened fluids orally. In two controlled studies the value of a gastric tube in slight cases did not become apparent. In severe cases a gastric tube facilitates monitoring of stress ulcer prophylaxis at a pH-optimum of 3–4.

Fluid replacement should amount to at least 3 l within the first 24 hours, however in moderate to severe cases it should amount to more, up to 6 l of electrolyte compound solutions. It is beneficial to maintain the fluid intake according to the central venous pressure. In the following days fluid administration including electrolytes, albumin and haemoglobin, as the case may be, is managed according to the rules of medical intensive care. Hypocalcemia always indicates hypoalbuminemia, on account of which albumin should be given additionally to calcium.

Impaired glucose metabolism is to be expected between the third and fifth day of the disease. When blood glucose levels exceed 200 mg % regular insulin is administered in relatively low doses at short intervals or as a continuous infusion. Parenteral hyperalimentation is not necessary in the early phase of acute pancreatitis and can increase the risk of catheter-induced septicemia. It is indispensable, however, in protracted cases, especially when local complications have arisen, or after surgery. Development of a paralytic ileus is not treated with prokinetic drugs such as prostigmin or caerulein as these drugs simultaneously stimulate pancreatic secretion.

Drugs

Analgesics

Analgesia is a primary aim in the treatment of acute pancreatitis, for one to cause subjective relief for the patient, for the other to reduce adverse reflective effects favoring hypovolemic shock. Several authors recommend a continuous infusion of procaine-hydrochloride, 2 g/24 h, as a basic therapy, although this measure has not been justified by controlled investigations. Regular administration of tramadole or buprenorphine and other morphine derivatives have proven their worth. Spasmolytics without analgesic components are ineffective and not indicated because of the accompanying intestinal paralysis. The analgesic effect of calcitonin has been confirmed by 2 studies. Further effect beyond pain relief in acute pancreatitis, however, could not be demonstrated.

Antibiotics are indicated in every case of biliary pancreatitis and in severe alcohol-induced cases. Biliary and pancreatic digestive drugs such as ampicillin, mezlocillin, cephalosporines and others are recommended.

Antisecretory drugs have no proven effect. Atropine is not indicated because of the adverse effect on the heart and circulatory system as well as intensification of intestinal paralysis. The polypeptides calcitonin, glucagon and somatostatin showed no effect in controlled studies. The proven analgesic effect of calcitonin is probably not due to beneficial influence on the course of acute pancreatitis, but possibly due to the liberation of endomorphines by this polypeptide hormone. Therefore an obligate recommendation to use calcitonin in acute pancreatitis does not exist.

H_2-blockers have no evident effect on the course of acute pancreatitis. They can, however, be employed in stress ulcer prophylaxis. Attention should be paid to the dosage, so that the pH is not raised higher than 4, as hereby the risk of pneumonia can increase due to bacterial colonization of the stomach and in case of gastropharyngeal reflux. Aprotinin (Trasylol®) is generally not very recommended. With exception of one study in England, no positive effect could be noted in a great number of studies.

Other enzyme inhibitors such as antifibrinolytics (EACA, AMCA or PAMBA) or phospholipase-A2-inhibitors such as procaine are also without confirmed value. The effectivity of synthetic protease- and phospholipase-A2-inhibitors Gabexat-Mesilat (Foy) are being tested in controlled clinical studies at present.

Endoscopic sphincterotomy (EST) is absolutely indicated in impacted prepapillary and intrapapillary calculi with extrahepatic bile obstruction. The diagnosis can be established by sonography. A relative indication for this measure exists when non-obstructive calculi of the bile duct are demonstrated by endoscopic retrograde cholangiography. Contrarily the indication is questionable in case of free bile drainage without evidence of stones in the main bile duct and evidence of uncomplicated stones exclusively in the gall bladder. The general indication to EST in acute pancreatitis stated by different authors in view of the concept of free drainage of the pancreas following opening of the papilla must be verified by controlled investigations.

Peritoneal dialysis – Haemodialysis

The rational reasoning behind peritoneal dialysis in the early stage of severe acute pancreatitis lies in elimination of toxic and vasoactive substances. The advantages of this measure observed in animal experiments could not be verified in clinical studies. In acute renal failure haemodialysis is indicated. This rarely becomes necessary, because as a rule, after the onset of renal failure the renal function recovers in time upon resolution of the acute episode of pancreatitis.

In protracted courses of the disease, which can be due to exacerbations or localized complications a catabolic metabolic state exists, making high caloric parenteral hyperalimentation necessary. It should be postponed in the case of pseudocysts, even with constantly elevated levels of pancreatic enzymes in the serum. In extreme pain and indication of superinfection immediate surgical intervention is necessary. Otherwise spontaneous regression within the next 3 to 6 months can be awaited before surgery becomes mandatory in the case of persistence.

3.3.6.2 Surgical Therapy

Although the acute necrotizing inflammation, with exception of biliary causes, can be controlled by conservative measures in most cases of clinically grade I acute pancreatitis, surgical intervention often becomes necessary under emergency conditions in grade III pancreatitis. Actual consideration of the indication and optimal timing for surgery is thus primarily necessary in grade II pancreatitis (Hollender et al 1983).

The indication for early surgery applies upon failure of conservative treatment, i. e. a progressive clinical deterioration of the patient's condition. The leading clinical symptoms during therapy inferred are: peritonitis, ileus, shock, progressive renal and respiratory failure, haemorrhages, coagulatory disorders, pancreatogenic ascites, intensification of jaundice (Hoffmann and Berthold 1979, Schalimov et al. 1980, Hollender et al. 1983).

There is extensive agreement as to the indication for early surgery in biliary pancreatitis. The smallest measure is elimination of duct compression by insertion of a T-drain. Bile duct revision can also be an indication for late surgery (Neher 1977). The indication may ensue upon progressive clinical deterioration of the patient's condition. This can be due to abscesses, larger sequesters, massive gastrointestinal haemorrhages. Computerized tomographic findings can give considerable support in establishing the diagnosis. By means of computerized tomography differential diagnosis of abdominal palpable tumors is possible due to their variable consistency. These may be abscesses, sequesters or pseudocysts. The pseudocysts initially do not constitute an indication for surgery, as even large pseudocysts can undergo spontaneous regression (Neher et al. 1980). Pseudocysts presenting clinical symptoms, however, definitely need surgical revision. According to present experience the moment for surgery should be delayed until the patient's condition is stable enough for therapeutic intervention.

Early surgery is related to high lethality. Ranson (1978) reported that 20 of 31 patients, who underwent surgery between the 1. and 7. day of illness died, in contrast to 102 patients, who were operated on after the 8. day of illness, of whom 18 died.

Of the surgical measures pancreatic operations and other surgical procedures must be distinguished from one another. Operations involving the pancreas itself are always necessary in grade II and III pancreatitis. Only the removal of the necroses can prevent systemic intoxication. The measures involving the pancreas include necrosectomy, which is generally performed by "digitoclasia" via a variably extensive lateral pancreatic resection including splenectomy as well as partial or total duodenopancreatectomy. Extirpation of the spleen has surgical-technical reasons for one thing, for another Schalimov et al. (1980) points out that the splenic blood vessels are often involved in the inflammation so that leaving the spleen increases the risk of uncontrollable postoperative haemorrhage. The extent of radicality is still a subject of controversy.

Table 9 Surgical measures in haemorrhagic-necrotizing pancreatitis (revised by Neher, 1977)

Clearing of necroses	
Resection (left lateral pancreatic resection, subtotal left pancreatic resection, duodenopancreatectomy)	
Clearing of peripancreatic channels of necrosis	
Drainage of the operation field	
Decompression of the bile ducts	
Cholecystectomy, Revision of the main bile duct, T-drainage	
Gastrostomy, Jejunostomy	
Drainage of Abscess	
Biliary Pancreatitis:	decompression of bile ducts, reconstruction of the bile ducts, transduodenal sphincterectomy

In view of possible long-term complications such as diabetes mellitus and malassimilation syndrome Fritsch (1980) prefers organ preserving techniques, which allow a layout of the resection preserving as much intact parenchyma as possible. Hollender (1983), on the other hand, prefers extensive resection, if possible, pointing out adverse results quo ad vitam and quo ad sanctionem in resection of the pancreatic head in necrosis of the same. Duodenopancreatectomy as the most radical measure, preferred by only few others, involves an often high lethality. This extensive operation is selected to reduce the general toxic effect of necrotizing pancreatitis. The high lethality occurring in those cases probably results from the high percentage of emergency surgery.

Extensive drainage of the operation site concludes each operation. Even peripancreatic necrotic tissue is drained. The remaining necrotic material is supposed to be flushed out via the drain. Hollender (1983) uses suction/flushing tubes. Peritoneal dialysis as a means of rinsing the abdominal cavity to remove inflammatory mediators has been propagated recently. Bücheler et al. 1985 point out that the lethality can not be significantly reduced by administration of peritoneal dialysis. In cases of peritoneal dialysis, however, a decrease in morbidity factors such as shock and organ failure can be reached. By means of a combination of necrosectomy and lavage of the Bursa omentalis especially retroperitoneal necrosis areas can be cleared better and results of surgical treatment improved.

Because of long-standing adynamic ileus gastrostomy and sometimes a nutritional jejunostomy are recommended in severe cases. Obstructional ileus, volvulus, abscess formation in vicinity of the stoma as well as uncontrollable diarrhoea can occur as complications of jejunostomy (Fritsch 1980).

Indications for surgery of the bile ducts must be seen in view of the etiologies of the diseases. In pancreatitis of biliary causes decompression of the bile ducts by drainage of the choledochal duct is mandatory. For corrective surgery of the bile ducts Hollender (1979) suggests a one-session, Kümmerle a two-session technique. Irrespective of the etiology Hollender (1979) and Schalimov et al. (1980) perform cholecystectomy and T-tube drainage to prevent bile obstruction, because in their opinion pancreatic oedema causes bile duct compression. This action is not accepted by Fritsch (1980) and other authors.

In severe cases of acute pancreatitis intestinal paralysis can arise owing to extension of the inflammation to the intestinal wall. Due to an increase in the intraabdominal volume the diaphragm is pushed upward. Compression of the thoracic space results in a restrictive ventilatory disorder. As the transverse colon is particularly affected and toxins from the large bowel can have adverse affects on the course of the disease, it is recommended to deal generously with the indications for an ileostomy (Horn 1983, Edelmann et al. 1985). More or less extensive bowel resections are occasionally necessary. In surgical therapy second operations must be reckoned with. New sequestration as well as abscess formation may make second operations necessary. Stenosis of the duodenum generally has a good prognosis and rarely makes gastroentero-anastomoses necessary (Klose et al. 1983). Fistula-formation out of granulation cavities as well as salivary fistula demonstrate a good tendency to spontaneous regression.

For some time laparostomy has been recommended in severest cases. The laparotomy remains wide open and is only covered by a foil. This measure allows for repeated peritoneal lavage. Possibly arising necroses can be removed daily. In adequate assessment of the indication this measure can improve the prognosis considerably in individual cases.

3.4 Chronic Pancreatitis (Figs. 51–63)

3.4.1 Definition

Chronic pancreatitis is a protracted inflammation of the pancreas characterized by a permanent alteration of the basic anatomical structure and thus frequent functional deficits, even if the cause is eliminated. In advanced stages a global reduction in function due to decreased exocrine and endocrine pancreatic function occurs.

3.4.2 Clinical Course

The clinical course of chronic pancreatitis depends on the stage of the disease at any given time and covers a highly acute condition presenting symptoms of an acute abdomen to high grade cachexia. The leading symptom is abdominal pain, occurring in 85% of the patients and experienced as low-situated, persistent, piercing or sharp (Forell 1979). In most cases the pain is diffusely localized in the upper abdomen and belt-like radiation to the back is considered typical, but not observed very often. Intensity of the pain attacks varies in case to case. Generally the pain succumbs only to opiates. The pain attacks in so-called alcohol-induced pancreatitis typically occur 12 to 14 hour after a drinking episode in patients with long-standing alcohol abuse (Marks et al. 1976).

Sudden pain, especially in later stages, also arises postprandially. The pain usually lasts for several days. In uncomplicated cases the symptoms subside after 3 to 7 days. Under the influence of persistent pain the patient resides in an antialgesic position in an attempt to find pain relief. The knees are pulled up to the chin, the fists are pressed into the upper abdomen. Even though intermittent pain attacks, interrupted by long pain-free intervals of up to several months duration represent the most common appearance, painless courses and such with persistent pain occur. According to Ammann (1987) the latter represent courses with local complications. In painless types symptoms arising from the exocrine and endocrine pancreas can be observed. Dyspeptic complaints such as persistent meteorism, the sensation of repletion, belching, food and stimulant incompatibilities, nausea and emesis also accompany the painful episodes. Occasionally the dyspeptic complaints occur prior to pain attacks, so that hours pass before a maximum is reached.

If pain attacks recur in short intervals many patients refuse nourishment out of fear of new episodes, so that weight loss up to 30% can take place. Massive foul-smelling greasy stools occur regularly in about 25 to 33% of the patients with chronic calcifying pancreatitis, indicating an advanced stage with pronounced malassimilation. It is to be reckoned with the occurrence of steatorrhoea 2 to 20 years after the manifestation of diabetes, which in turn follows the first pain episode in 5 to 10 years (Marks 1976, Ammann 1987). "Kwashiorkor"-like pictures with hypalbuminemic oedema, wrinkling and discoloration of the skin and hair have been described in few individual cases (Sarles 1976, Marks 1976).

Inhibited, depressive or fearful, agitated moods can be observed in chronic pancreatitis (Colmant and Noltenius 1977). The term "pancreatic encephalopathy" coined by Rothermund (1941) summarizes the large number of neurologic and psychopathologic findings. In 14 to 19% of the cases with pancreatitis neuropsychiatric peculiarities can be observed on an average 3 to 5 days following the onset of pancreatic symptoms. Apart from increased proprioceptive reflexes, generally without pyramidal signs, an increase in the tonus of the extremities and nuchal musculature, delirious, hallucinatory, paranoid and comatose forms, which are often accompanied by hyperthermia are seen, especially in acute phases. Endocrine functional disturbances of the pancreas become clinically apparent due to impaired glucose tolerance. Retinopathy, nephropathy and arteriosclerosis are rarely complications, probably because of the long time spans necessary for their development (Marks et al. 1976). Increased fluctuation of blood glucose levels, especially causing problems in alcoholics in the postoperative period following total duodenopancreatectomy, takes on special significance, as regular food intake and elimination of alcohol are not guaranteed. Apart from the symptoms typical for longstanding pancreatitis manifold symptoms of acute pancreatitis occur in acute exacerbations, such as violent pain localized in the middle of the epigastrium in 70%, radiating to the left or right depending on the localization. In 80% of the cases emesis accompanies the pain. In 50% a moderate, in 15% a severe state of shock develops, which can be complicated by functional ileus (in isolated involvement of the transverse colon, so-called Goblet-Guyon-sign) or pulmonary dysfunction. In 15–20% localized left pleural effusion or atelectasis and ensuing respiratory failure must be reckoned with (Ammann 1987).

Due to the topographic relationships the duodenum, colon, splenic vein and portal vein are the neighboring organ structures endangered by pancreatitis. Thrombosis of the portal and splenic veins become apparent not only by haematemesis and melaena. The pathogenesis of pancreatogenic ascites is associated with segmental portal hypertension with hypalbuminemia. Pancreatic cysts appear to have chief significance in the genesis of pancreatogenic ascites. In more than 2/3 of the cases with pancreatogenic ascites "leaks" in the form of ruptured pseudocysts and open pancreatic ductal lesions are found (Hotz 1978).

Pseudocysts are of causal significance for stenoses of the duodenum and colon because of their massive character. Even though most stenoses of the colon subsequent to pancreatitis are incomplete and are based on pancreatic intercrescence, total obstruction, necroses of the colon with ensuing perforations or fistula as well as spontaneous ruptures of pancreatic pseudocysts into the bowel have become known (Lankisch et al. 1976). Leading symptoms are, apart from colic-like upper abdominal pain, increasing constipation and rectal passage of blood. In these cases differential diagnosis includes gastrointestinal ulcers, whose frequency is reported as 2 to 19% in alcohol-induced pancreatitis, thrombosis of the splenic vein, gastric erosions and Mallory-Weiss-syndromes. A characteristic allowing differentiation is the time of occurrence. Postoperative haemorrhage can ensue from tryptic arrosion of the blood vessels. Haemorrhages, which are associated with an acute episode are due to prehepatic portal hypertension or gastritis. Interval haemorrhaging is more frequent in association with a gastric ulcer or bleeding varices (Marks et al. 1976).

3.4.3 Diagnostics (Figs. 51–55)

The clinical diagnosis "chronic pancreatitis" is based on anamnestic data, the physical, radiologic, sonographic, endoscopic and laboratory chemical findings. Purpose of the various examination methods is obtaining evidence and establishing of the extent of the morphologic damage, or as the case may be, obtaining evidence of endocrine or exocrine functional disturbances. An exact diagnosis, however, can be established only about 5 years following the first episode presenting typical clinical symptoms (Ammann 1987). Especially in uncomplicated cases the history of the longitudinal course can thus result in an early suspicion and represents the basis of further diagnostic measures. In planning the technical investigations orientating measures during the symptom-poor interval should be taken into consideration in the interest of expedience and in order to go on to special examination procedures.

The screening tests (Table 10) can offer clues as to the etiology of chronic pancreatitis (hypercalcemia, hyperlipoproteinemia). They can also give indications as to regional complications (Gamma GT, Bilirubin). Whereas serum amylase and especially serum lipase levels are elevated especially in parotitis, liver diseases and renal failure, during acute episodes or complications, low cholesterin-, albumin- and electrolyte concentrations in the serum or, as the case may be, a reduced prothrombin index, may be indicative of an advanced stage of malassimilation (Forell 1979).

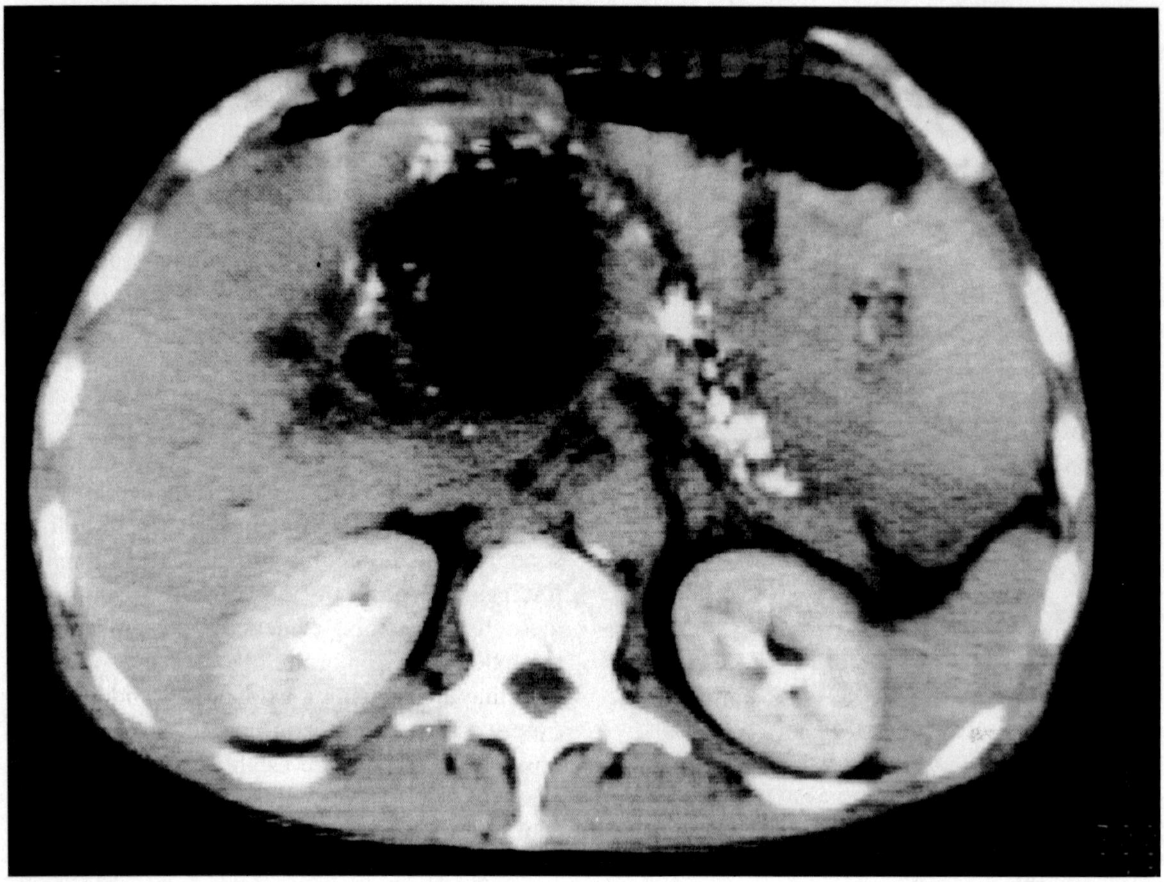

Fig. 51
Computerized tomograph. Acute episode of chronic pancreatitis with calcium-dense structures in the pancreatic tail area and large necrosis in vicinity of the pancreatic head with sequestration into neighboring organs.

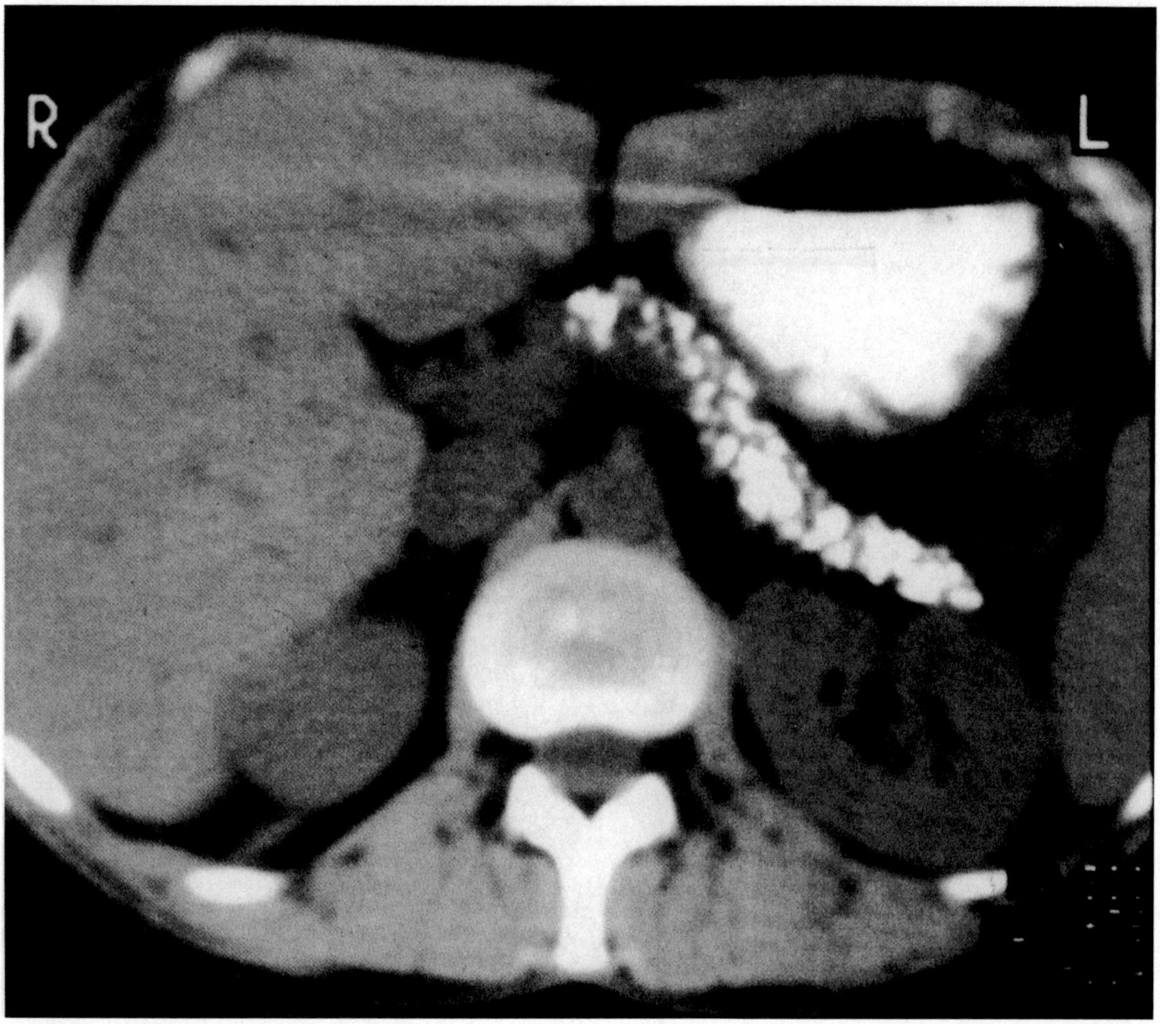

Fig. 52
Computerized tomograph in chronic pancreatitis. Calcification and multiple calculi in the corpus and tail area.

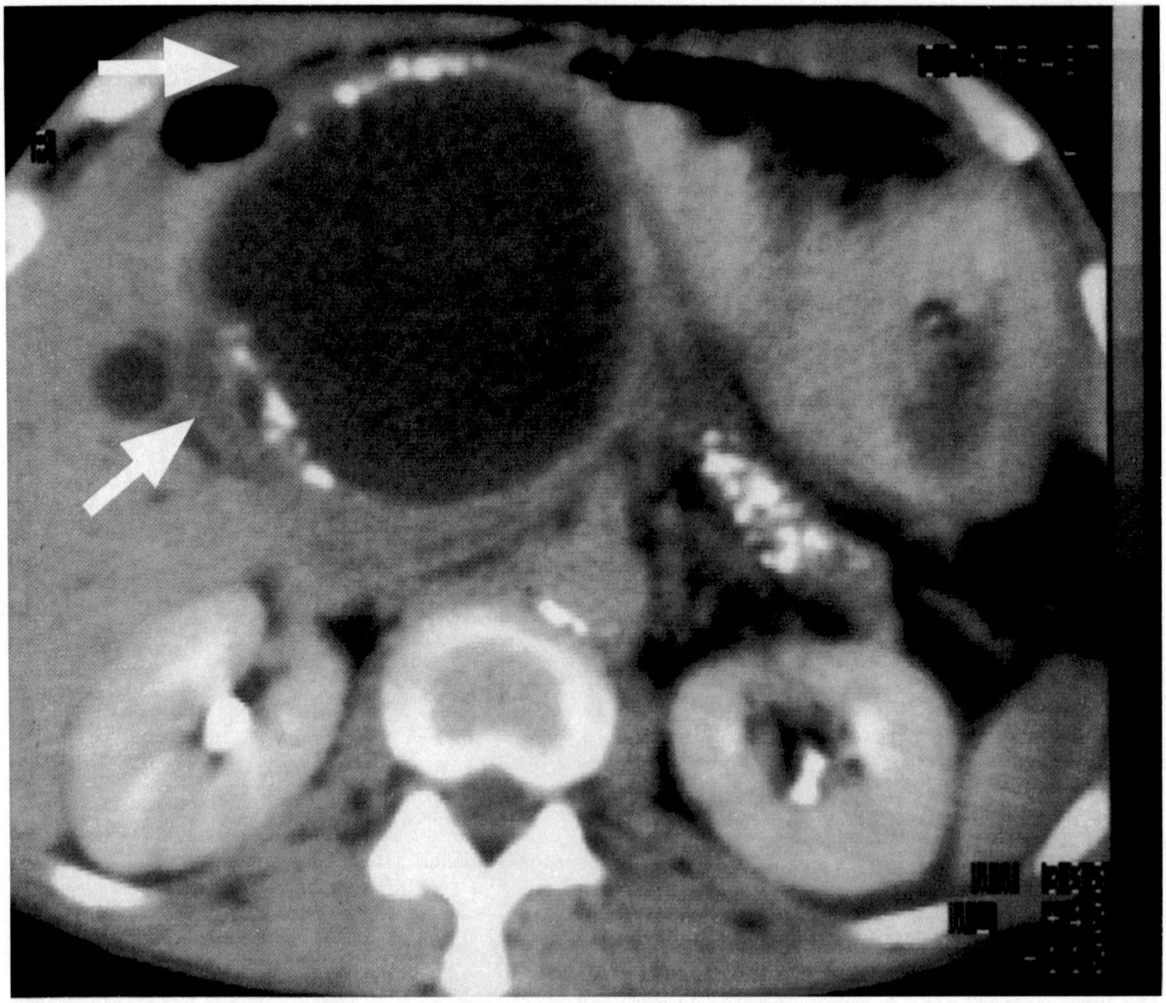

Fig. 53
Computerized tomograph. Large pancreatic pseudocyst in the head area with calcifications in the cyst wall. Adjacent calcifying pancreatitis in the tail area.

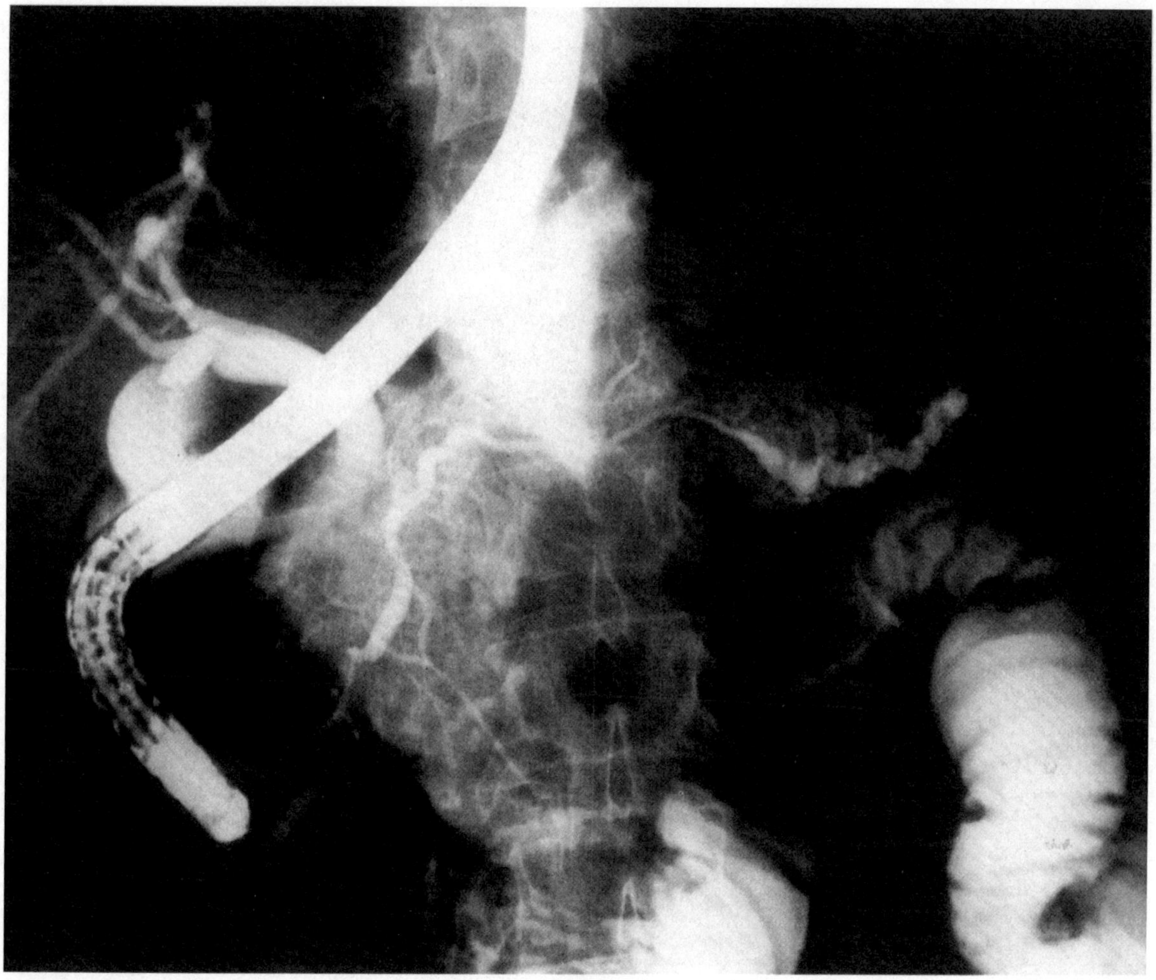

Fig. 54
Endoscopic retrograde cholangiopancreatography in chronic pancreatitis. Choledocholithiasis with stenosis of the papilla. Chronic pancreatitis with irregular course of the duct (stenoses) in the tail area.

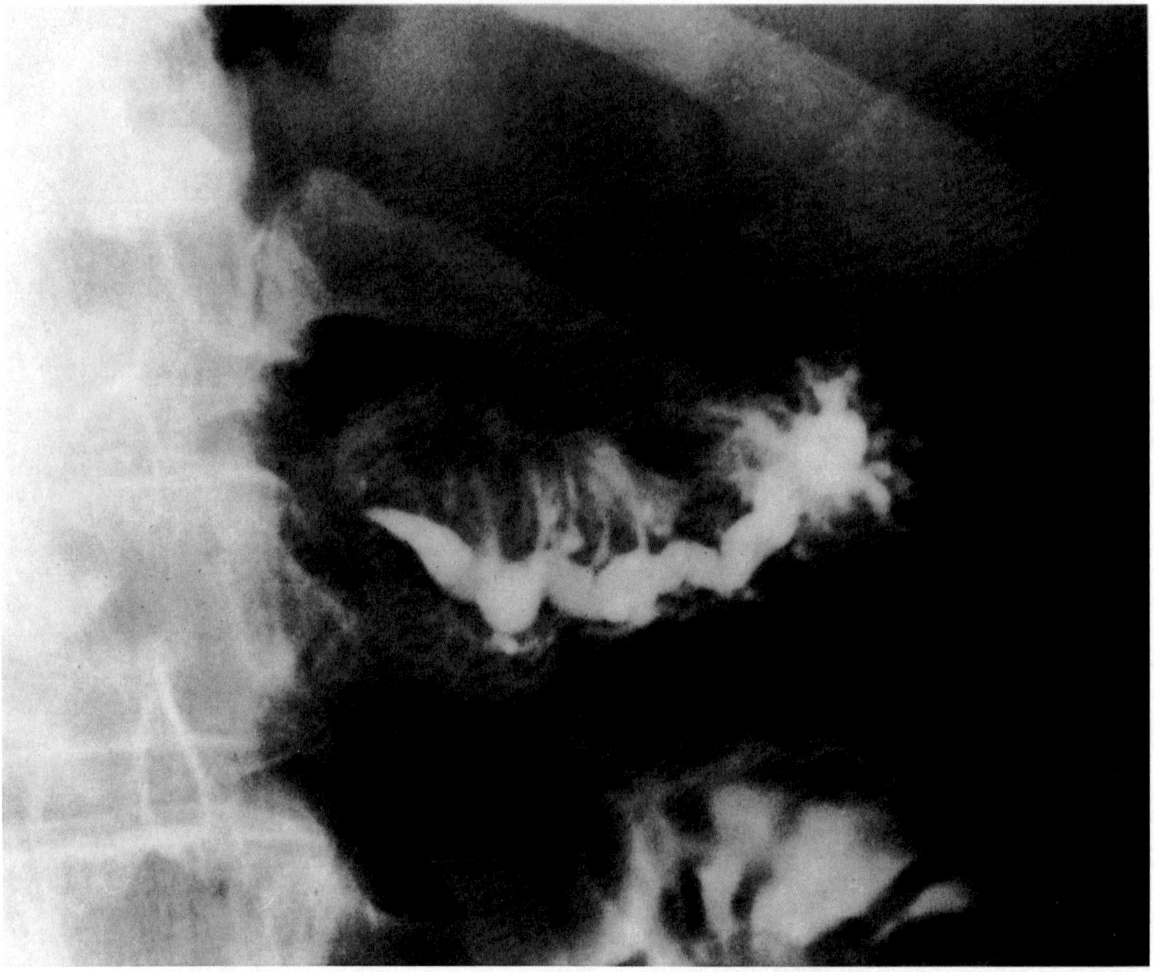

Fig. 55
Endoscopic retrograde cholangiopancreatography in chronic pancreatitis. Marked dilatation of the ductal system with irregularly distributed stenoses.

Table 10 Screening tests (mod. by Forell 1979)

- *Laboratory examinations:*
  lipase, amylase, trypsin-RIA, Gamma GT, alkaline phosphatase, bilirubin
  Ca^{++}, blood fat content, glucose metabolism, prothrombin index
  D-Xylose-Test
  Chymotrypsin in the Stool
  PABA-Test
  van der Kamer (quantitative estimation of fatty acids)
  Vitamin A-tolerance test
  weight of stool
- *Sonography of the upper abdomen*
- *Radiographic examinations:*
  upper gastrointestinal x-ray series
  upper gastrointestinal x-ray series with duodenography
  I. V.-cholecysto-, cholangiography
  preliminary abdominal radiography
- *Oesophago-gastro-duodenoscopy*

Table 11 Direct and indirect procedures to test exocrine pancreatic function (mod. by Lankisch et al., 1984)

1. Direct tests of pancreatic function
   - Secretin-pancreatozymin test
   - Lundh test meal
2. Indirect tests of pancreatic function
   a) Measurement of an enzyme
      - trypsin in the stool
      - pancreatic-isoamylase in the serum
      - immunoreactive trypsin in the serum
   b) Measurement of an enzyme performance
      - NBT-PABA-test
      - quantitative stool fat determination (according to van de Kamer)
   c) Measurement of a pancreatic hormone
      - pancreatic polypeptide

The examination procedures pertaining to the function of the pancreas serve to assess the secretional capacity of the organ. Direct and indirect methods must be distinguished from one another (Table 11). The most reliable direct method is the secretion-cholecystokinin-pancreozymin test (S-CCU-Test), which has a success rate of 90%. The principle of the test is based on analysis of the pancreatic secretions following hormonal stimulation of the hydrokinetic and ecbolic function of the pancreas. In view of the necessity to acquire intraluminal pancreatic secretions via a double lumen gastroduodenal tube and the difficulty of standardization, the test is only available to few examiners. Oral stimulation by a test meal (Lundh-Test) does not make the complicated method any easier. The NBT-PABA and the pancreolauryl tests are available as indirect tests. Both methods demonstrate sufficient sensitivity and specificity, but involve a certain degree of effort due to the 6 to 10 hourly urine collection period in order to measure the paraaminobenzoic acid or respectively its fluorescence (Lankisch et al. 1984).

Examination methods developed so far, which are easy for the patient to perform, attain only a low degree of sensitivity and specificity in comparison to direct functional tests. Steatorrhoea is not to be expected until later stages of chronic pancreatitis when more than 75% of pancreatic tissue has been resected or is reduced to 10% of the norm owing to lipase secretion (Otte 1979).

Determination of chymotrypsin in the stool has been found to be a practical detector test. A sensitivity of 78% and specificity of 84% can be expected due to easily accessible examination material capable of arbitrary repetition and easy biochemical analysis (Lankisch et al. 1984). One disadvantage in the method lies in the lower sensitivity in slight to moderate exocrine pancreatic insufficiency.

The remaining known pancreatic function tests have – with exception to the evaluation of the endocrine situation with aid of oral glucose stimulation – not been generally accepted for clinical use. The significance of newer methods such as assay of pancreatic polypeptides and immunoreactive trypsin remain to be seen. Progress in regard to distinction of inflammation- from tumor-induced pancreatic insufficiency is not to be expected from these methods either (Malfertheiner et al. 1984).

Diagnostics of the morphology of the pancreas encounter difficulties due to the "hidden" location of the organ. With computerized tomography, sonography and ERCP 3 special methods are available to evaluate the pancreatic parenchyma. The usual conventional methods of x-ray examinations have their place in preliminary diagnostics. Calcifications are found in spot radiography of the pancreas in up to 60% of advanced cases. Complications such as ileus and left pleural effusion are also registered. The application of special morphologic examination methods depend on the advantages and disadvantages of the techniques. ERCP has established itself as the most precise method in diagnosis of chronic pancreatitis and differentiation from pancreatic carcinoma (Gmelin 1981). It is true that ERCP also determines inflammatory parenchymal lesions only indirectly via secondary alterations of the ductal system, however, first alterations can already be demonstrated in the side branches. The value of ERCP lies in the demonstration and precise evaluation of alterations eligible for surgery. Combination with cytological examinations can enhance the differential diagnosis of pancreatic carcinoma, contributing to establishing the optimal moment for possible surgical intervention (Arendt et al. 1979).

If only little time is left to prepare for elaborate methods and moreover, if infiltration of the pancreatic surroundings has taken place and a topographic-anatomic overview is needed, performance of a computerized tomographic scan of the abdomen is the obvious method to choose. Difficulties with excessive intraluminal intestinal gas or adipositas, as in 10 to 20% of the cases, where the pancreas cannot be depicted by sonography, pale into insignificance. However, sonography has established itself as an unstrenuous screening method for sequential monitoring of the course of the disease. The pancreatic pseudocysts can be depicted especially well by sonographic examinations because of the typical echo pattern. Problems in classification ensue only in differentiation of haematomas and pseudocysts, especially in the pancreatic tail area (Huck et al. 1981). Excluding the less important morphologic examination methods (e.g. pancreatic scintigraphy, laparoscopy) the tabular overview (Table 12) summarizes the characterisitics of the different methods available for diagnosis of chronic pancreatitis.

Table 12 Morphologic examination methods – Characteristics of chronic pancreatitis and accuracy

1. Sonography
- swollen, enlarged, echo-poor pancreas
- fibrotic, small pancreas lacking outer contours and with irregular echos within (in "difficult" interval)
- fibrotic, small pancreas lacking outer contours and with irregular echos within (in "difficult" interval)
- highly intense reflections indicative of calcifications (Dammann et al., 1982)
- dilatations of main bile duct and pancreatic duct (Botzler et al., 1981)
- good demonstration of cysts larger than 1 to 2 cm in diameter (Bücheler et al., 1982)
- easy follow-up of the course of the disease

Accuracy (mod. by Büchler et al., 1985)

Examiner	n	correct	incorrect	indefinite
Sheedy II	20	70%	20%	10%
Fiegler	33	70%	30%	
Gmelin (1981)	19	68%	21%	11%
Lackner (1980)	113	70% (sensitivity)		

2. *Computerized tomography (Lackner et al. 1980, Büchler et al., 1982)*
   - organ enlargement and deformation with dispersal of the organ structure
   - calcifications larger than 1 to 2 mm in diameter
   - pseudocysts
   - advantage of practicability in adipose patients and existing meteorism
   - opportunity for application of intravenous contrast medium increases yield of further diagnostic information

   Accuracy (mod. by Büchler et al., 1985)

Examiner	n	correct	incorrect	indefinite
Sheedy II	20	85%	10%	5%
Haaga	19	68%	32%	
Fiegler	33	85%	15%	
Pistolesi	48	64%	6%	30%
Moss	21	62%	33%	5%
Gmelin (1981)	19	84%	5%	11%
Lackner (1980)	113	84% (sensitivity)		

3. *ERCP*
   - distension and stenosis of the duct of Wirsung
   - structural alterations of the minor ducts
   - intraductal calcifications
   - taking contraindications into consideration it applies to wait for a period of 3 to 4 weeks after an acute episode has subsided
   - pseudocysts are considered a contraindication as acute pancreatitis with sepsis ensues in 90% of the cases upon filling of the cyst, 20% of the cases taking a lethal course
   - it is reckoned with a complication rate of 1 to 3% at a mortality rate of 0.2% (Forell, 1979; Otte, 1979; Tympner et al., 1979)
   - complication prevention includes avoiding parenchymal dyeing procedures
   - diffuse ductal alterations are not to be expected before manifest secretory dysfunction is evident

   Accuracy (mod. by Büchler et al., 1985)

Examiner	correct	incorrect	indefinite
Lit. overview	83%	6%	10%
Gmelin (1981)	89%	11%	0%

4. *Angiography*
   - evidence of stenoses and dilatations of prepancreatic arteries
   - vascular dislocation owing to enlargement of the pancreas
   - variation of areas with increased and decreased vascularization
   - pronounced meandering of veins (Dammann et al., 1982)

   Accuracy (mod. by Büchler et al., 1985)

Examiner	correct	incorrect	indefinite
according to citation in Büchelor (1982)	50–85%		

5. *Conventional radiographic methods*

5.1 *Abdominal x-rays*
   - left-sided shadowing of the costo-diaphragmatic recessus
   - calcification of the pancreatic region, verified by spot radiography, confirms the diagnosis
   - level formation in the upper jejunum
   - lacking collection of intestinal gases in the transverse colon, so-called Stuart's colon-cut-off-syndrome
   - displacement of the lienal flexure (Klemm, 1979)

5.2 *Upper gastrointestinal barium meal, hypotonic duodenography*
   - impressions, displacements and infiltrations allow indirect conclusions about mass lesions
   - varices of the gastric wall in stenoses of the splenic vein or the root of the portal vein
   - simulation of a gastric or duodenal ulcer
   - watering-can-phenomenon in the duodenum, possibly also biconcave configuration (Frostberg's sign) or evidence of stenosis of the duodenum or a diverticulum
   - marked alterations of the pancreatic head easily demonstrable in hypotonia (Forell, 1979)

5.3 *i. v. cholangiography*
   - owing to nonspecific alterations of the main bile duct only limited application

3.4.4 Prognosis of Chronic Pancreatitis

By means of long-term studies with an average observation period of over 10 years Ammann (1987) developed a staging in chronic pancreatitis. In uncomplicated courses 3 stages can be distinguished.

In stage 1, which is characterized by a typical attack of pancreatitis of days to approximately one week duration, alternating with an interval free of complaints lasting months, morphologic alterations can not be registered with the aid of apparative methods. In the large group of alcohol-induced pancreatitis the average age of the patients concerned is 36.2 years. Especially men are affected, the age span reaching from 19 to 63 years. After 5.5 years manifest endocrine and exocrine insufficiency sets in and announces transgression to stage 2. Aside from pathologic results in the pancreozymin-secretin test and decreased glucose tolerance calcifications can be demonstrated in up to 70% of the cases radiologically by pancreatic spot radiography. Clinically pain episodes are less pronounced at this stage. The frequency of the pain episodes diminishes. In stage 3a complete burn-out of the gland develops in an average of 6.8 years. At this point the clinical signs of severe global pancreatic failure are prime features. Manifest diabetes can be observed in 1 to 12 years after the first pain attacks (Dammann et al. 1982).

An association between the diabetes of chronic pancreatitis and the occurrence of pancreatic calcifications is typical. 50% of non-calcifying, but 90 % of the calcifying types show pathologic glucose tolerance. Pronounced lability with characteristic hypoglycemic states occurs. The course of the illness can be complicated by uncontrollable states of pain, which not infrequently lead to addiction of morphine (narcotics).

Life expectancy and the general condition of the patients with chronic pancreatitis after surgical treatment depend not only on the etiology of the disease and selection of the surgical procedure, but are also influenced considerably by the patients' cooperability in readjusting their lifestyles (Kozuschek et al. 1986).

Following extensive resections the patients exhibit a reduction in working capacity of 60 to 100%, however reintegration into the working process should be strived for. Inspite of the increase in the number of manifest diabetics from 52 to 82% subsequent to surgical treatment of pancreatitis and mandatory enzymatical substitution, extensive resections with according adjustment of the life style is tolerated well (Kümmerle et al. 1979).

Table 13 Follow-up of patients with chronic pancreatitis (Rösch et al., 1981)

Therapy	Subjective improvement		Lethality	
	after 3 years	after 7 years	after 3 years	after 7 years
conservative	71%	47%	8%	22%
resectional	72%	47%	20%	33%
non-resectional	62%	44%	24%	36%
	n = 348	n = 322	n = 348	n = 322

Fig. 56
Surgical specimen after standard Whipples's operation for chronic calcifying pancreatitis with lithiasis. In the extremely distended parts of the ductal system irregularly limited calculi (arrows). Adjacent an indistinct lobular structure of the parenchyma with broad, gray white scarred zones.

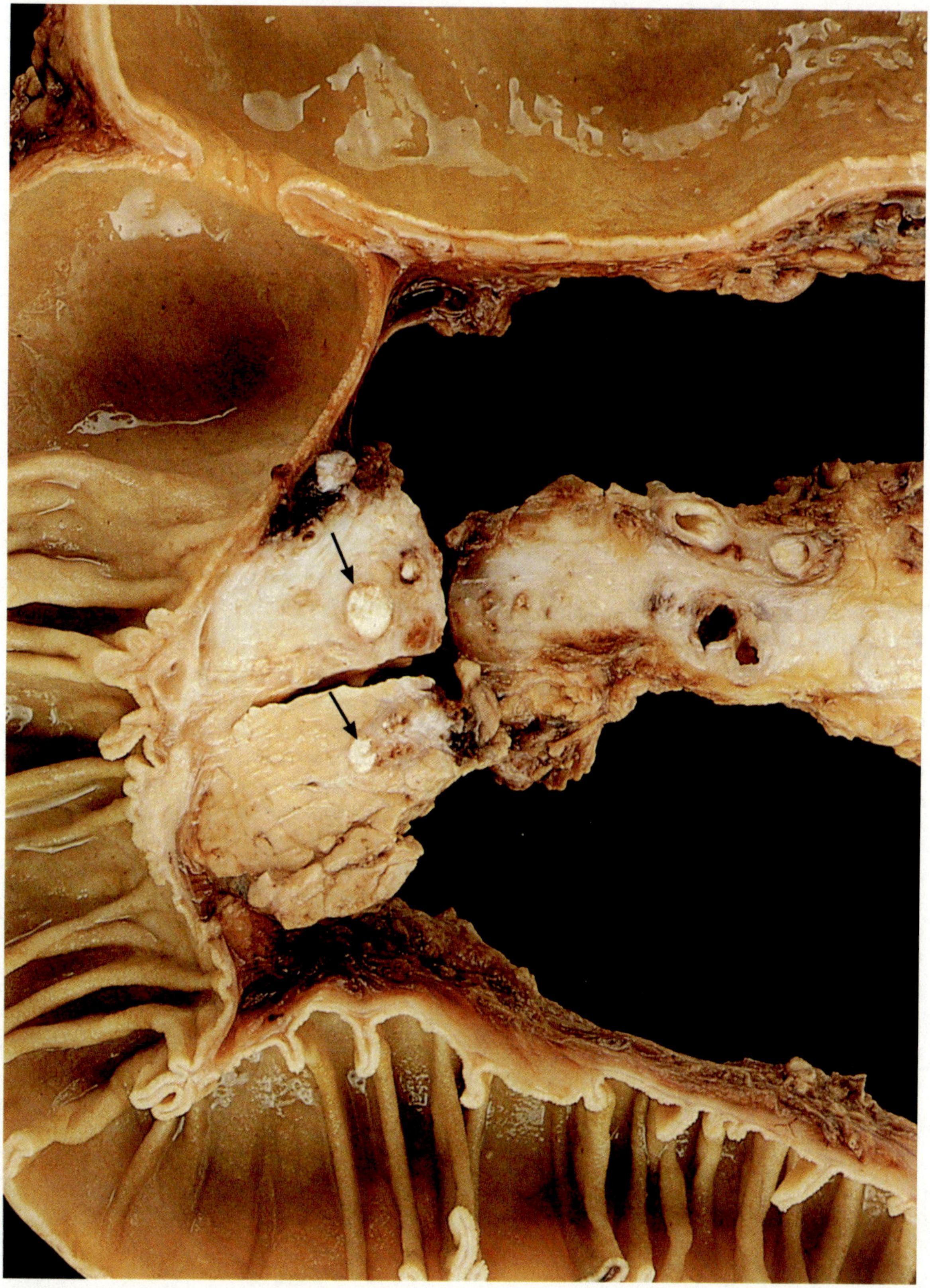

3.4.5 Morphology of Chronic Pancreatitis (Figs. 57–69)

Morphology of chronic pancreatitis is characterized by a progressive, scarred reconstruction of the exocrine parenchyma of the gland (Stolte 1987). According to extent and distribution of the scarring the following forms can be distinguished:

1. chronic pancreatitis with diffuse or segmental fibrosis
2. chronic pancreatitis with or without focal necroses
3. chronic pancreatitis with or without calcification
4. chronic obstructive pancreatitis.

Chronic pancreatitis with diffuse or segmental fibrosis

Stolte (1987) suggested adding specifications as to the extent of the scarring to the Marseille Nomenclature, in which the degree of severity remains unconsidered in respect to the classification.

In keeping the following can be distinguished:
Grade I = slight scarring
Grade II = moderate scarring
Grade III = high grade scarring
Grade IV = complete scarring.

Slight scarring shows a predominantly perilobular arrangement and extends into the lobuli in a moderate degree. In grade III chronic pancreatitis the initially still limited intralobular scars display confluence forming larger areas. In grade IV considerable scarred reconstruction with almost complete destruction of the exocrine parenchyma has taken place.

The extent and composition of the cellular inflammatory infiltrate is dependent on the degree of fibrosis. In slight scarring there is also only a slightly developed infiltrate composed of lymphocytes, plasma cells and scattered macrophages. In pronounced scarring only slight lymphocytic infiltrates can be demonstrated.

In the case of protracted fibrosis reactive fibrosis of the intima of arteries and arterioles develops, the extent of which follows the degree of fibrosis. The islets of Langerhans exhibit relatively few alterations in light microscopy, whereas Klöppel et al. (1978) could demonstrate a relative decrease in B-cells and increase in A-cells by electron microscopy. Only in advanced stages is a more prominent reduction of the islets to be reckoned with due to perivascular fibrosis of the intrainsular capillaries.

The ductal system is dilated in increased scarring. Increased convolutions and calibre variations of the ducts arise. In the scarring process folding of the lamina propria ensues from the formation of new fibres, resulting in reduced drainage of the secretions (Stolte 1987). The epithelium in the dilated ducts flattens. Papillary epithelial hyperplasia and squamous epithelial metaplasia can arise regionally. Depending on the degree of scarring protein-rich secretion plugs can be demonstrated in the dilated ducts, mainly in the tributaries to the smallest side branches of the duct of Wirsung. Probably as a result of inspissation of the secretions calcifications can develop in the ducts.

The alteration of the structure of the ductal system forms an essential requirement for the protracted course of the disease. The increasing reduction in drainage of secretions ensuing from fibrosis and epithelial damage in the ducts are responsible for limiting the protective functions of the ductal epithelium, so that continuous influence of the pancreatic secretions on the tissue constituents becomes possible. A vicious circle is upheld, which can be held responsible for the progressive scarring in the inflammatory condition.

According to systematical studies of Stolte (1987) chronic pancreatitis occurs in about 40% of the cases as segmental fibrosing pancreatitis. In this form the scarring is distributed irregularly, focally. More severely scarred areas alternate with relatively unaltered areas. Even the secondary alterations of the vessels and in the ductal system correspond with this segmental arrangement of the scarring and match the alterations that can be observed in diffuse fibrosis.

The alterations of the acinar cells depend on the degree of scarring. In the inflammation induced by alcohol abuse drops of neutral fat are evident in variable distribution in the cytoplasm. Fat inclusions, limited by a simple membrane, can confluate to larger drops of fat measuring up to 5 μm in diameter. Variable activity in respect to secretion production and exocytosis occurs. The number of zymogen granula located at the apical pole of the cell can be extremely decreased. Cells showing only scanty prosecretion granula or none at all can be found next to cells displaying active secretion production, although the endoplasmic reticulum appears unchanged. In areas of advanced fibrosis an irregular loosening of the endoplasmic reticulum also develops. Variably large autophagolysosomes, which can contain concentrically layered osmiophilic membranes and lumpy material, develop in the cytoplasm. Relatively large intracytoplasmic cavities filled with variably dense, granular material, can also be observed. They measure up to 5 μm in diameter and some lie adjacent to the basal and lateral cell membranes. Free connections between the cavities and the intercellular spaces may develop.

Similar vacuolar structures can be observed in caerulein-induced experimental pancreatitis (Kern 1987). The vacuoles form by fusion of the condensed vacuoles and zymogen granula in the Golgi region so that large cavities filled with proteinaceous secretions develop. The vacuoles and zymogen granula can fuse with the basolateral cell membrane and empty their contents into the intercellular spaces and interstitium. These findings indicate that chronic pancreatitis is probably maintained by protracted, misdirected secretion and release of secretions into the acini.

A reduction in the number of the cells in the acini occurs. The intercellular spaces between the acinar epithelium open up, so that free connections between the acinar lumen and the periacinar connective tissue zones arise. Individual cell necroses arise in the acini. The centroacinar cells belonging to the ductal system exhibit hydropic swelling of the cytoplasmic matrix. Variably large drops of neutral fat are evident in the cytoplasm.

The epithelium flattens in the dilated efferent ducts. Pronounced degenerative changes take place in the epithelial cells. They are characterized by a swelling of the cytoplasmic matrix and the cell organelles. Mucous production is highly reduced. Variably large and dense secretion complexes lie in the dilated ductal lumina. In the broad, scarred areas irregularly intertwined collagen fibre fascicles are developed. The scar tissue is only slightly vascularized. Only scattered lymphocytes and macrophages with relatively large phagolysosomes can be found in the fibrous structure.

The remains of the ducts and acini enclosed in the scarred areas consist of variably large cells with cellular nuclei varying greatly in shape, so that the differential diagnostic distinction between degenerately altered parenchymal residues and carcinoma can be difficult.

3.4.6 Therapy of Chronic Pancreatitis

The treatment of chronic pancreatitis is a subject of controversy. This is due to the great number of factors influencing the individual course of chronic pancreatitis, thus making individual therapy mandatory. Spontaneous courses and the incidence of complications differ depending on the collective of patients, so that a clearly defined, generally acknowledged strategy in the therapy of chronic pancreatitis does not exist.

Three principles of treatment are presented (Hoffmeister and Trede 1982):
- diet avoiding nutritive noxas, particularly alcohol
- treatment of endocrine and exocrine insufficiency
- pain control and correction of pancreatic complications.

Chronic pancreatitis represents an autonomic, variably progressive, chronic inflammatory condition at the moment of diagnosis. A causal therapy with the aim of complete restitution is not possible. The inflammatory process can be restrained in its dynamics if the causative agent can be eliminated. This applies especially for alcohol, which repre-

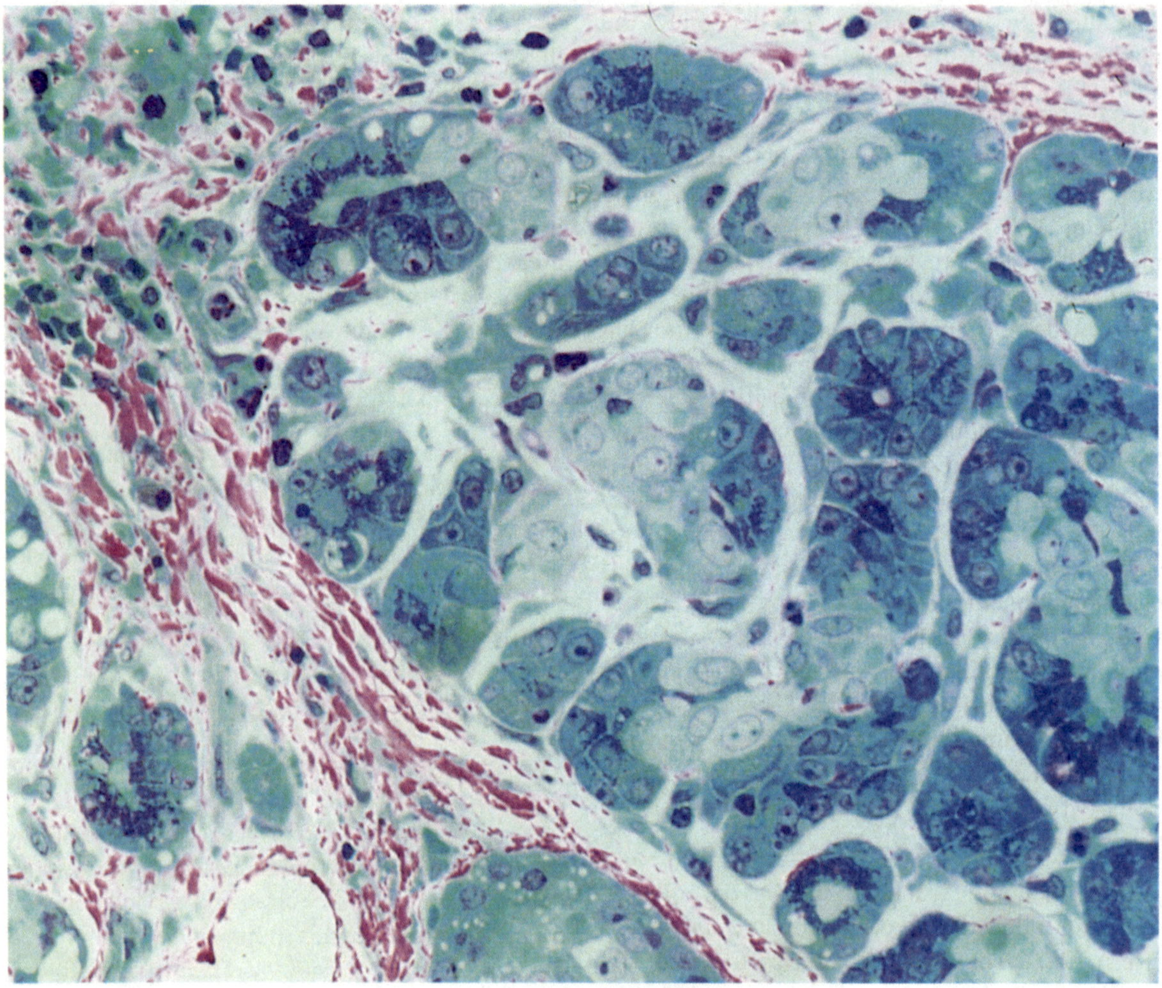

Fig. 57
Chronic pancreatitis with segmental fibrosis. Perilobular arrangement of concentric fibrosis, which develops in variably broad fibrous fascicles, extending into the individual lobuli. Interstitial oedema in the lobuli. Variably pronounced reduction in secretory activity of the acinar epithelial cells. Oedematous swelling and enlargement of the centro-acinar cells.
Light micrograph
Semithin section
Stain: Basic fuchsin and methylene blue
Magnification: 640 ×

Fig. 58
Fatty degeneration of the acinar cells in chronic pancreatitis. Between the lamella of the endoplasmic reticulum and scanty mitochondria variably large confluating neutral fat inclusions (arrows). ▷
Transmission electron micrograph
Magnification: 19300 ×

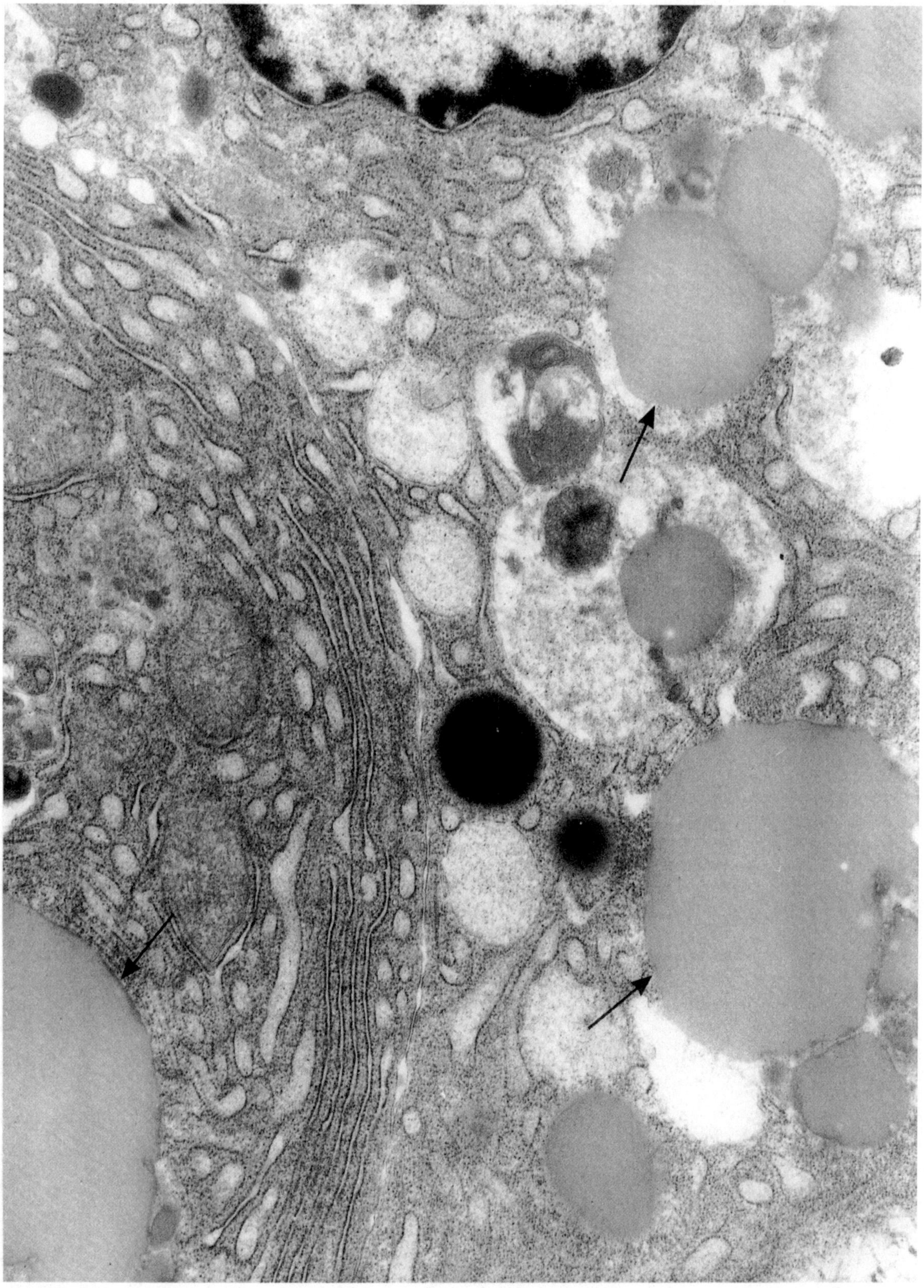

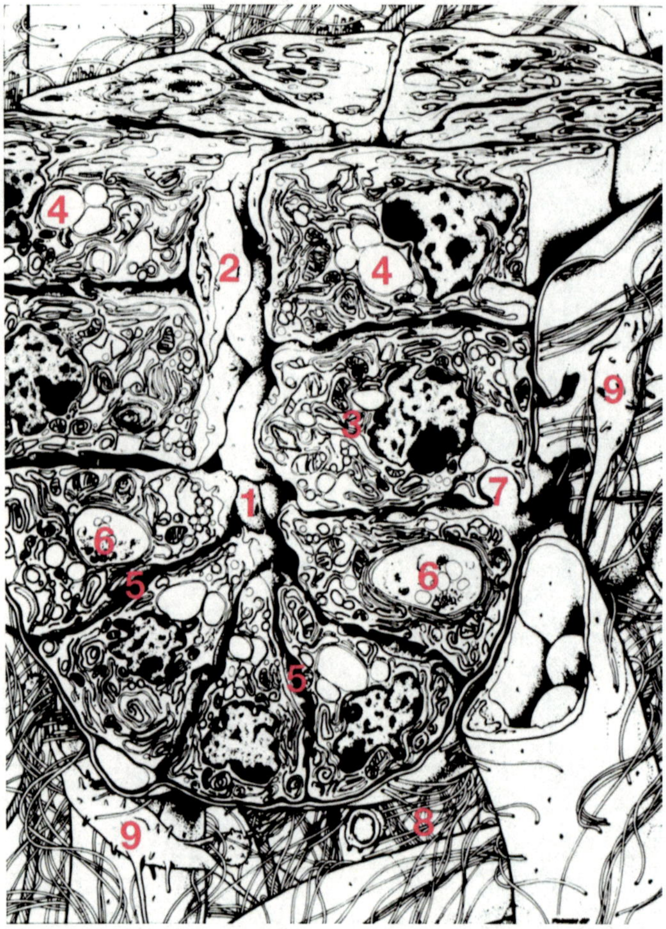

Fig. 59
Alterations of the acinar epithelial cells in chronic pancreatitis. Three-dimensional reproduction. Dissolution of the epithelial association with marked distension of the intercellular spaces. Open connection between acinar lumen and interstitial connective tissue. Variably marked vesicular transformation of the endoplasmic reticulum. Swelling and loosening of the mitochondria with shortening of the mitochondrial cristae. Formation of variably sized autophagolysosomes with partially granular, partially laminar contents. Defects in the basal lamella. Interstitial fibre formation.

1. acinar lumen
2. centro-acinar cells
3. oedematous, swollen acinar cell with distension of the endoplasmic reticulum
4. neutral fat inclusions
5. distension of the intercellular spaces
6. autophagolysosomes
7. migration of zymogen granula beyond the basolateral portions of the acinar cell to the interstitium
8. interstitial fibrosis
9. activated fibroblasts

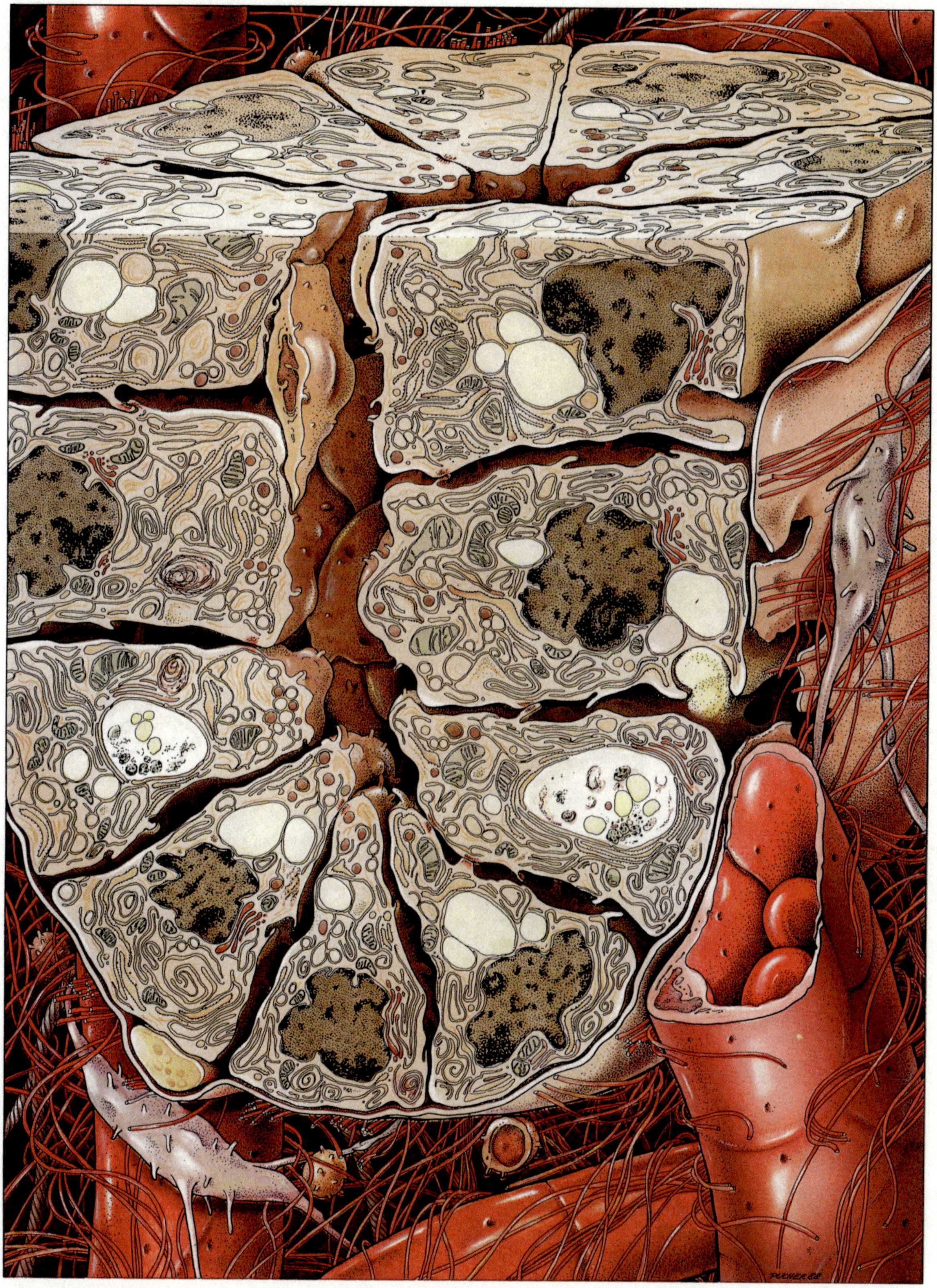

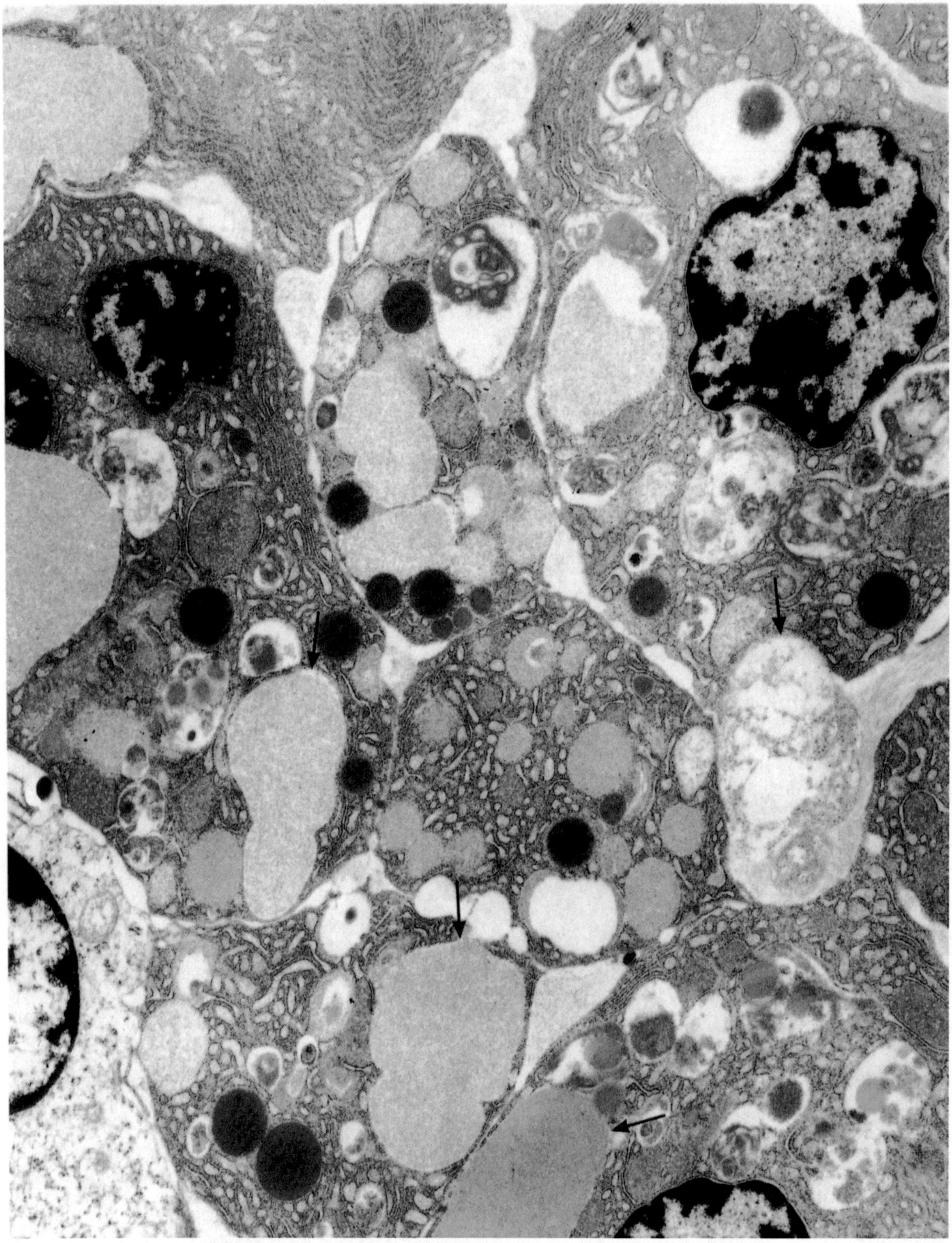

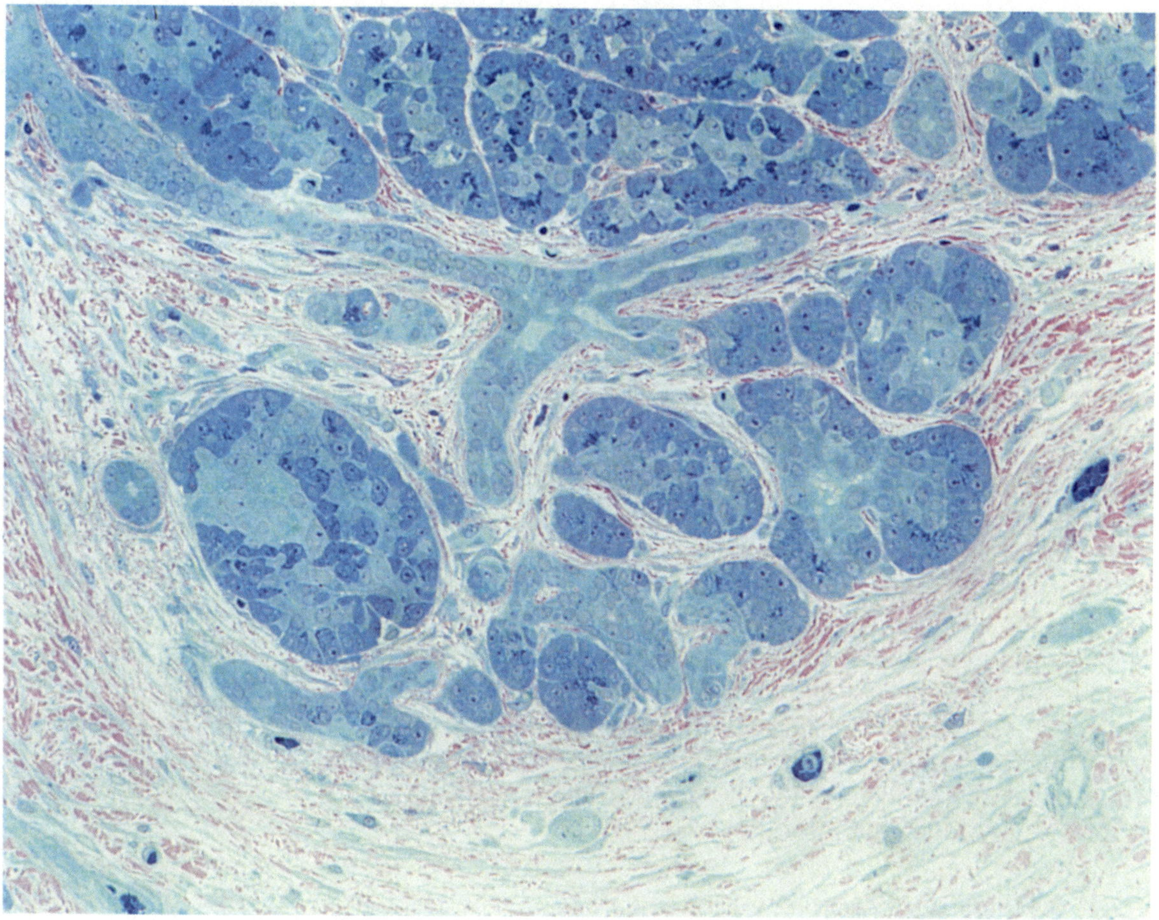

◁ Fig. 60
Alterations of the acinar cells in chronic pancreatitis. Variably marked shrinkage of the cellular nuclei. Irregularly distributed zymogen granula in the cytoplasm. Formation of variably large vacuoles with fine granular contents (arrows). Variable large autophagolysosomes with partially layered, partially amorphous material.
Transmission electron micrograph
Magnification: 8200 ×

Fig. 61
Advanced interstitial scarring in chronic pancreatitis with diffuse fibrosis. Marked atrophy in the pancreatic parenchyma. Individual acini are enclosed in broad fibre zones. Marked reduction in secretory activity. Terminal branches of the ductal system with pronounced periductal fibrosis. In the scarred zone only scanty lymphocytes and macrophages.
Light micrograph
Semithin section
Stain: Basic fuchsin and methylene blue
Magnification: 390 ×

sents the primary cause in more than 90%. In the rare cases arising from other causes these must be identified and be eliminated, if possible. This applies particularly to surgical revision of the bile ducts in biliary genesis or the rare case of primary hyperparathyroidism. Hence the essential aims of therapy of chronic pancreatitis are primarily the elimination or treatment of the consequences of the chronic inflammation with exocrine and endocrine insufficiency. Alcohol withdrawal, which essentially determines the prognosis of the disease both in respect to conservative measures as well as the success of surgery must be focussed on.

Patients with chronic pancreatitis before or after an operation for pancreatitis must be subjected to careful follow-ups regularly. Attention must be paid to stabilization subsequent to alcohol withdrawal on the one hand and the development of local complications possibly requiring surgery or not infrequently occurring concomitant diseases such as tuberculosis and carcinoma of the lung or oesophagus on the other. The physician must also engage in aiding professional and social rehabilitation (Table 14 and following presentation).

Table 14 Aims of therapy in chronic pancreatitis

- Alcohol withdrawal
- Freedom of pain
- Substitution in exo- and endocrine insufficiency
- Recognition and treatment of concomitant diseases
- Professional and social rehabilitation

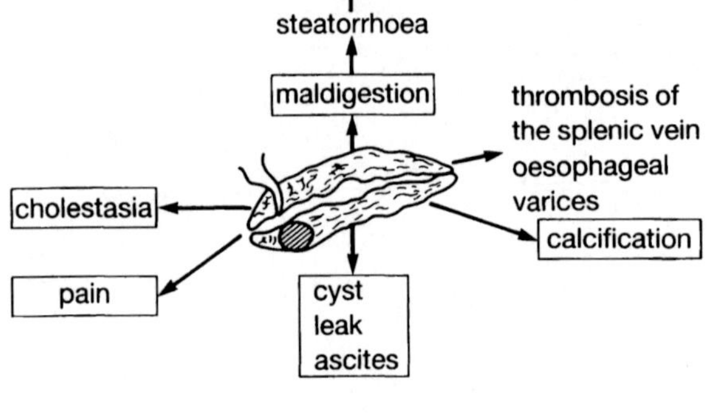

Pathophysiology of chronic pancreatitis as approaches to therapy

Fig. 62
Excessive distension of the intercellular spaces in the acinar system in chronic fibrosing pancreatitis. Open connection between acinar lumen and periacinar connective tissue. In the intercellular spaces fine granular material. In the adjacent cytoplasm of the acinar epithelial cells irregularly distributed zymogen granula with marked distension of the endoplasmic reticulum.
Transmission electron micrograph
Magnification: 10000 ×

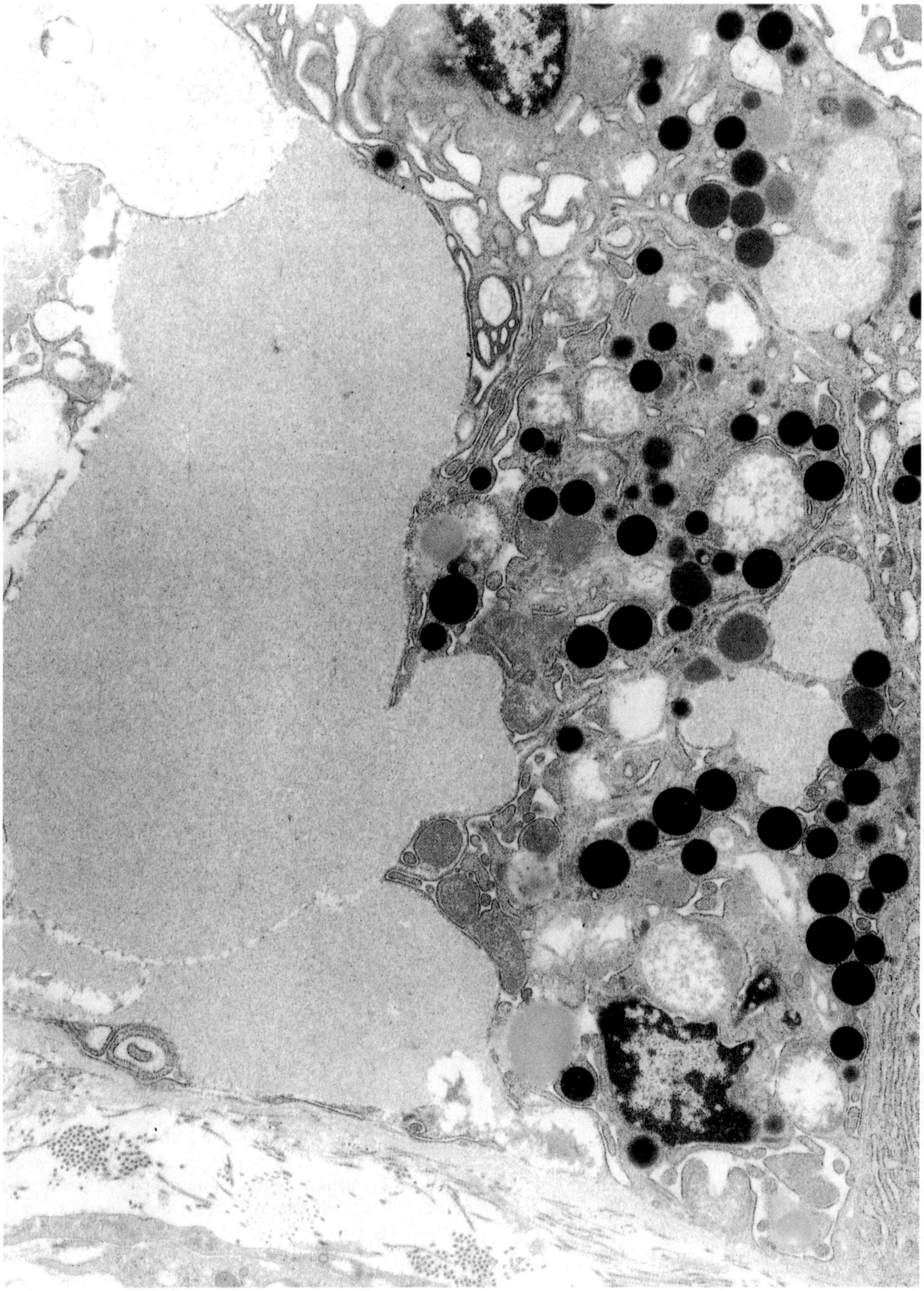

3.4.6.1 Conservative Treatment

General measures (Table 15): Regular follow-up and talks with the patient are imperative for clinical and social stabilization. In cases of pertinent alcohol dependency family members must be included and the possibilities of Alcoholics Anonymous, psychotherapy and if necessary psychiatric treatment must be called upon. A social worker should be consulted.

Table 15 General measures in chronic pancreatitis

1. Elimination of noxes (alcohol abstinence, surgical correction of the bile ducts, etc.)
2. Regular follow-up and talks (including relatives)
3. In alcohol addiction: Alcoholics Anonymous (AA)
   psychotherapy
   psychiatric treatment
4. Resocialization (social worker)
5. Diet: frequent small meals (2500–3000 cal/d)
   adequate pancreatin substitution
   reduction of fats to 60 g/d: 540 kcal
   in severe cases addition of MCT 80–120 g/d: 660–1000 kcal
   carbohydrates: 300–400 g: 1200–1600 kcal
   adjustment of insulin dose, if necessary
   protein: 60–120 g: 320–480 kcal
   in cachexia and anorexia elementary diet via gastric nutritional tube.

Diet: Owing to frequently marked catabolism and maldigestion patients with chronic pancreatitis should receive a total of more than 2500 calories. The prescription of a strict fat-free diet is considered obsolete at present. Easily digestible vegetable oils are tolerated well and do not aggravate the chronic inflammatory condition or postprandial complaints. Especially on account of the high caloric content dietary fats are indispensable. An addition of the middle-chained triglycerides is only necessary in severe states of maldigestion and severe malnutrition resistant to treatment; due to the bad taste and the complicated preparation it can be dispensed with as a rule. Carbohydrates should be offered in abundance even when manifest diabetes mellitus is present. Higher molecular polysaccharides should be given preference. The protein intake should amount to 80 to 120 g/d in the form of easily digestible foodstuffs such as milk products, eggs, tender meat and fish. A high caloric elementary diet or even parenteral hyperalimentation is only indicated in severe cachectic, anorexic stages, often accompanied by localized complications, e. g. prior to planned surgical intervention.

In conclusion it applies that the fare must be an easily digestible, balanced diet acceptable in taste for the patient, possibly under additional enzyme substitution.

Substitutional Treatment (Table 16)

Table 16 Substitutional treatment in chronic pancreatitis

Pancreatic enzymes
- ▶ early indication in pain
- ▶ late indication in malabsorption

Insulin (oral antidiabetics useless)
- ▶ correction with sufficient CHO-intake (300–400 g CHO)
- ▶ Desired blood glucose level: 120–180 mg% (CAUTION Hypoglycemia!)

Fat-soluble vitamins (-A, -D, -K)
- ▶ parenteral substitution only in severest terminal stages

Fig. 63
Marked degenerative alterations of the acinar epithelium in chronic pancreatitis. In the cytoplasm small droplets of neutral fat. Formation of large autophagolysosomes (arrows). Adjacent partially layered, lamellar and contrast-rich amorphous material.
Transmission electron micrograph
Magnification: 6400 ×

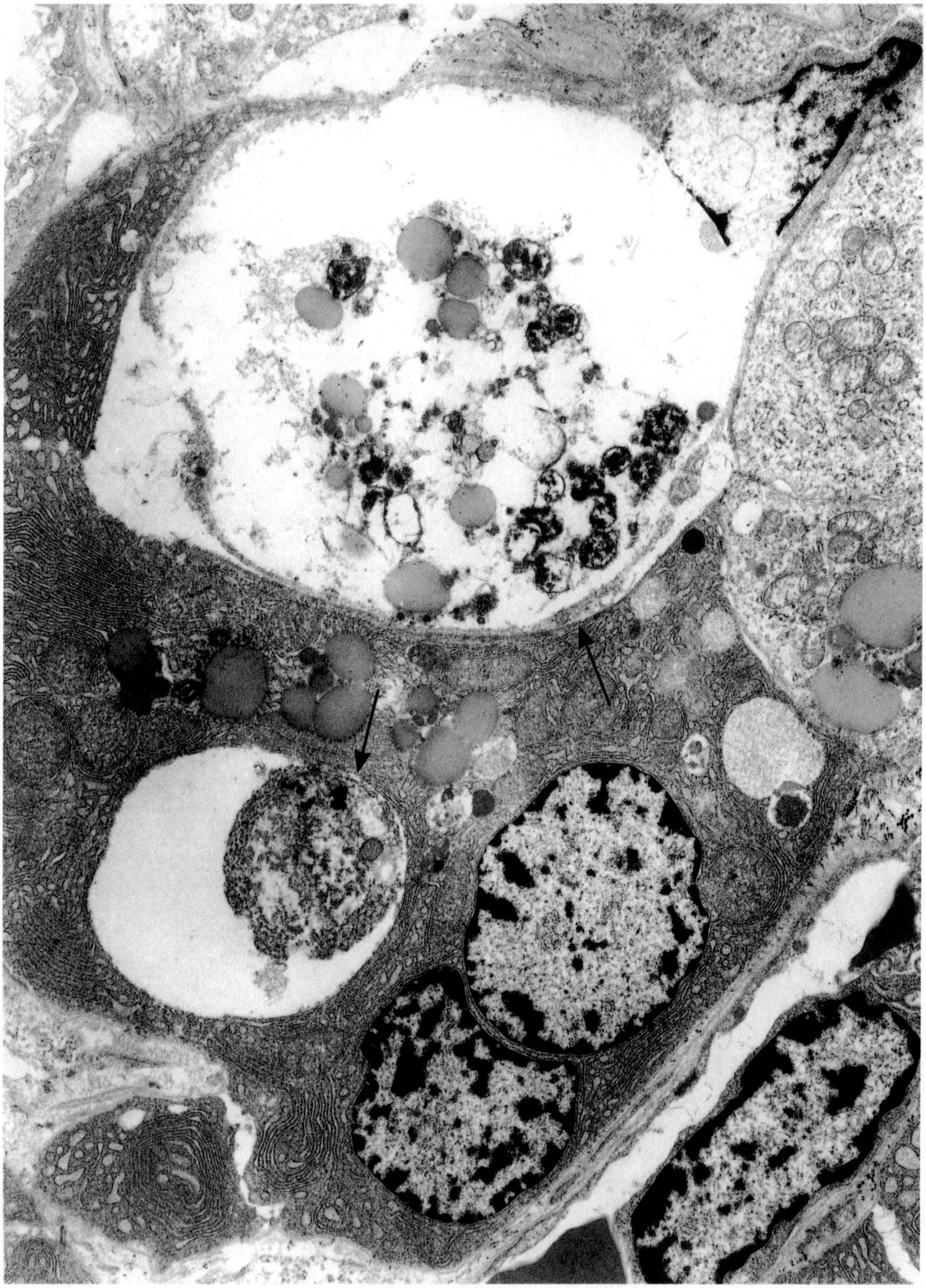

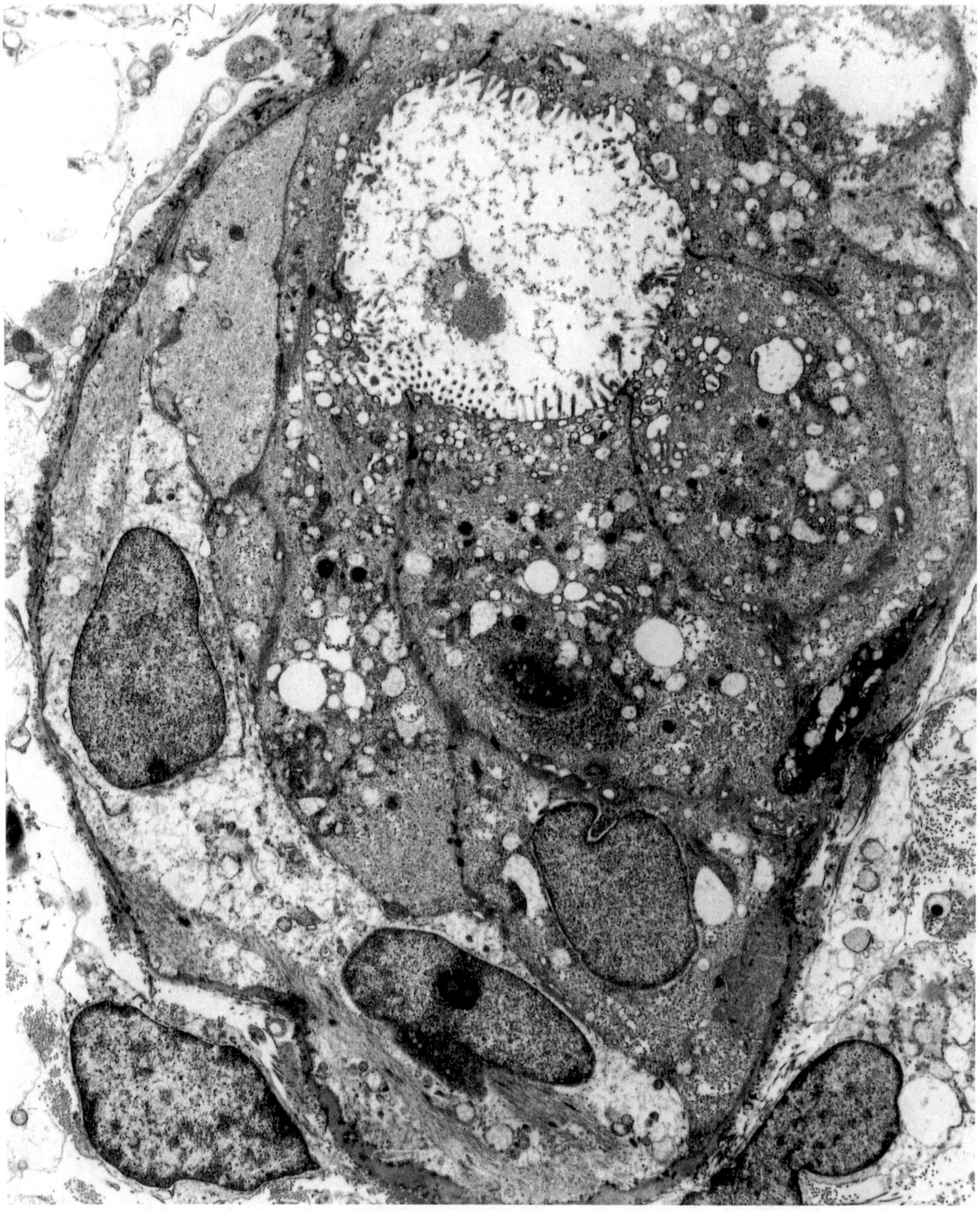

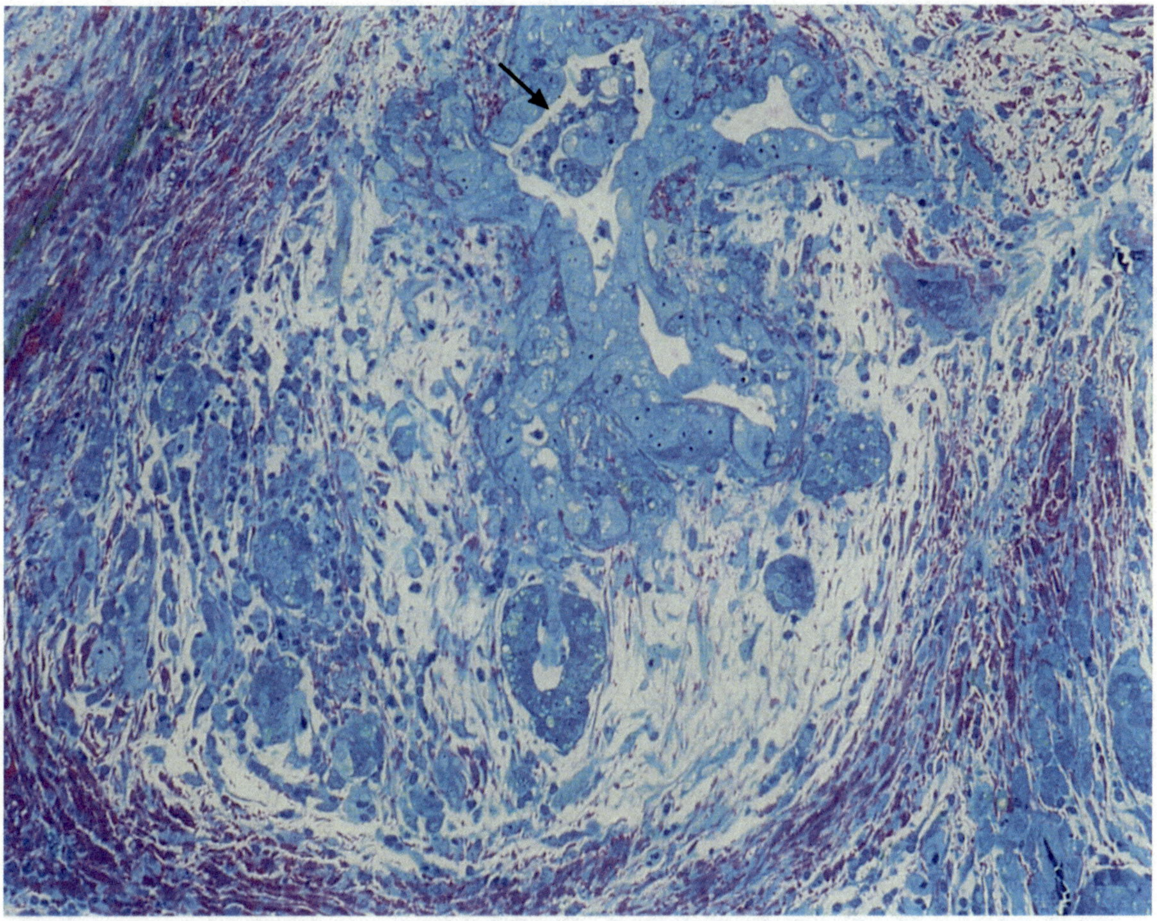

◁ Fig. 64

Residuum of a terminal branch of the ductal system in advanced fibrosis of chronic pancreatitis. Intact microvilli structure at the surface of the epithelial cells. Vesicular distension of the endoplasmic reticulum and vesicular transformation of the mitochondria in the ductal epithelial cells. Variably marked oedematous dispersion of the cytoplasmic matrix of the ductal epithelium.

Transmission electron micrograph
Magnification: 5200 ×

Fig. 65

Extreme atrophy of the acinar system in chronic pancreatitis with profuse scarring (grade III). In extensively scarred areas only traces of the terminal branches of the ductal system are maintained. In the ductal lumina focal small zones of proliferating epithelium (arrow). Slight lymphocytic infiltration in the scars.

Light micrograph
Semithin section
Stain: Basic fuchsin and methylene blue
Magnification: 390 ×

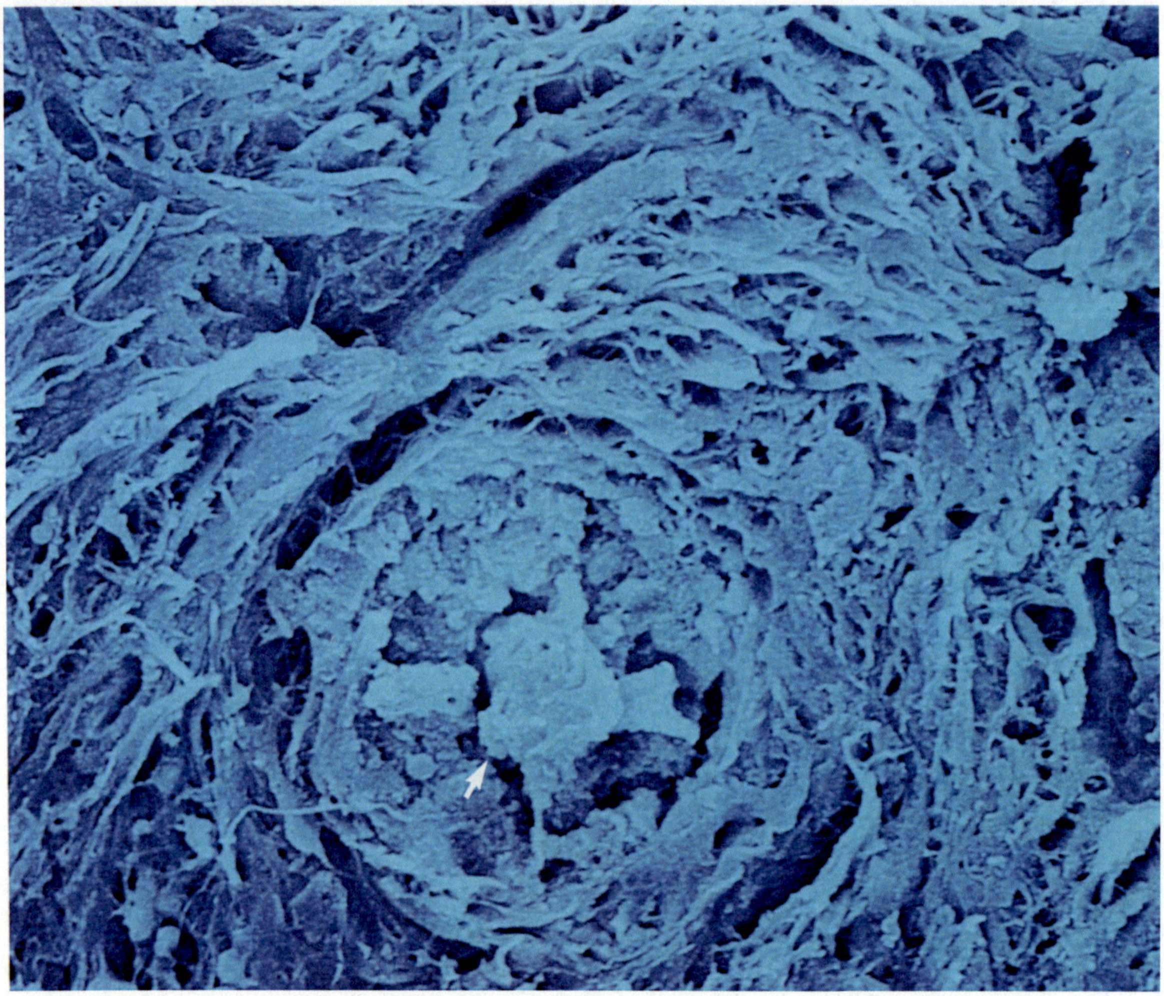

Fig. 66
Advanced scarring in chronic pancreatitis with diffuse fibrosis enclosing ductal residuum. In the ductal lumen exfoliated epithelial cells and secretion complexes (arrow). Surrounding the duct concentrically arranged fibre zone with course, irregularly interlaced tracts of collagen fibres.
Scanning electron micrograph
Magnification: 720 ×

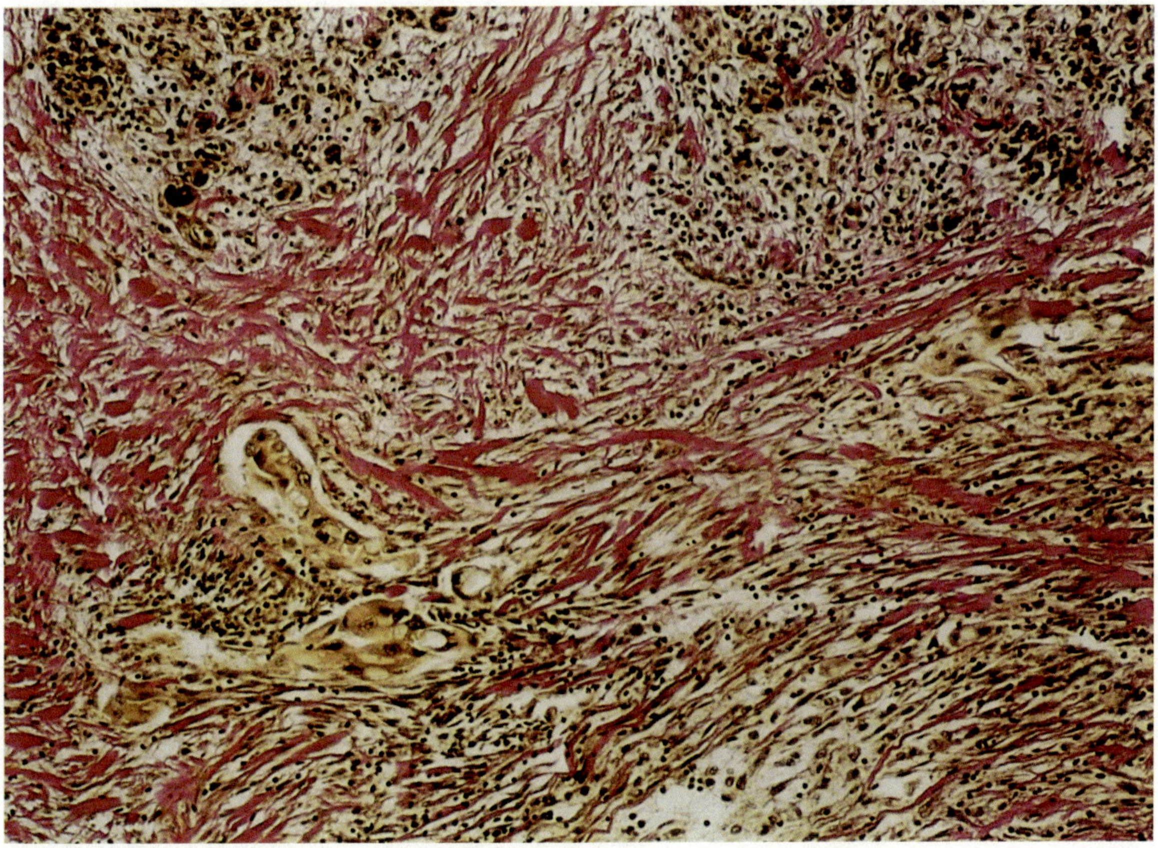

Fig. 67
Advanced fibrosis in chronic pancreatitis with extreme atrophy of the glandular parenchyma. In the broad collagen fibre-rich, scarred zones only residua of the ductal and acinar systems. In the fibrosis slight infiltrates with lymphocytes and scattered macrophages.
Light micrograph
Stain: van Gieson
Magnification: 210 ×

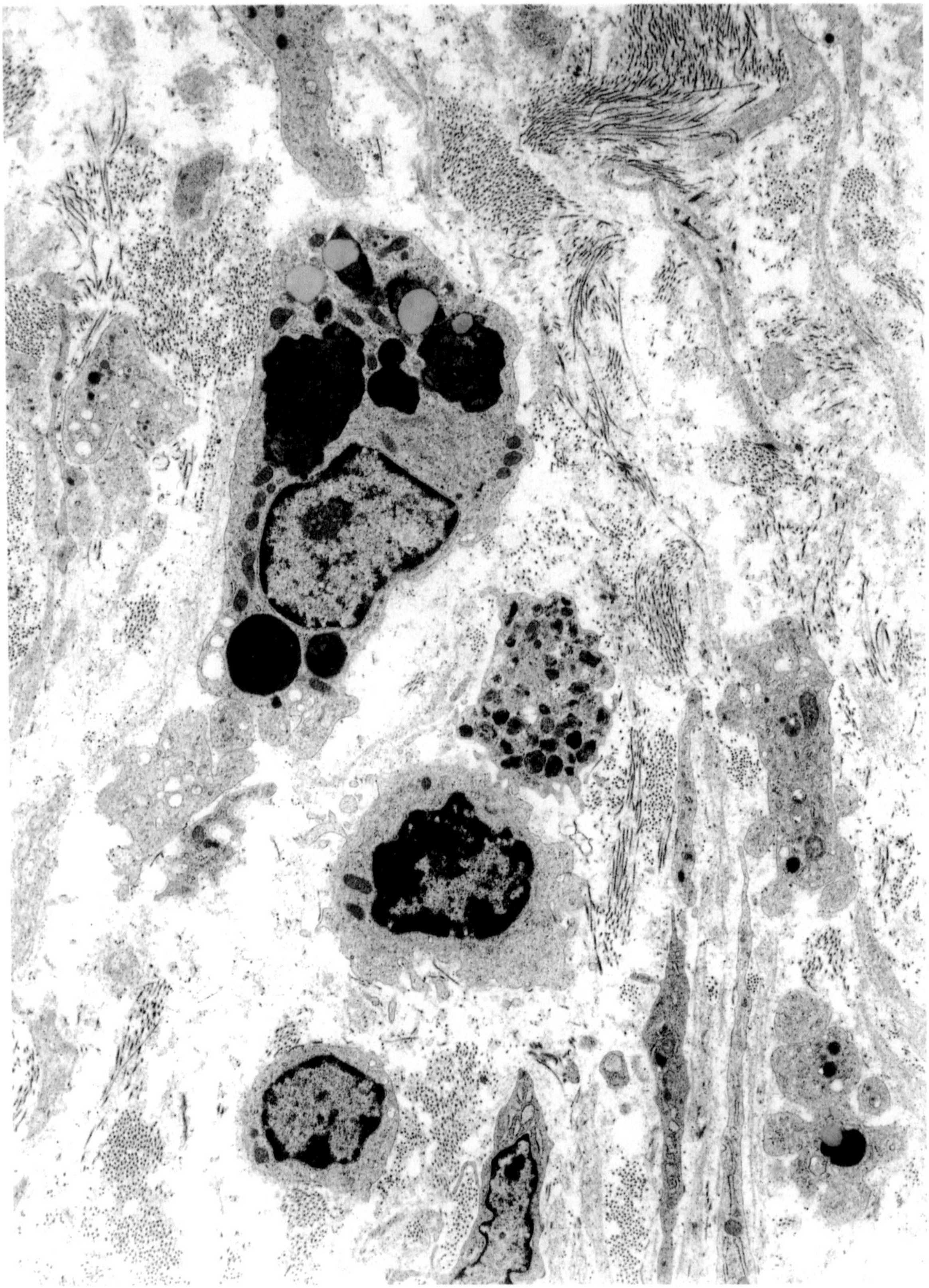

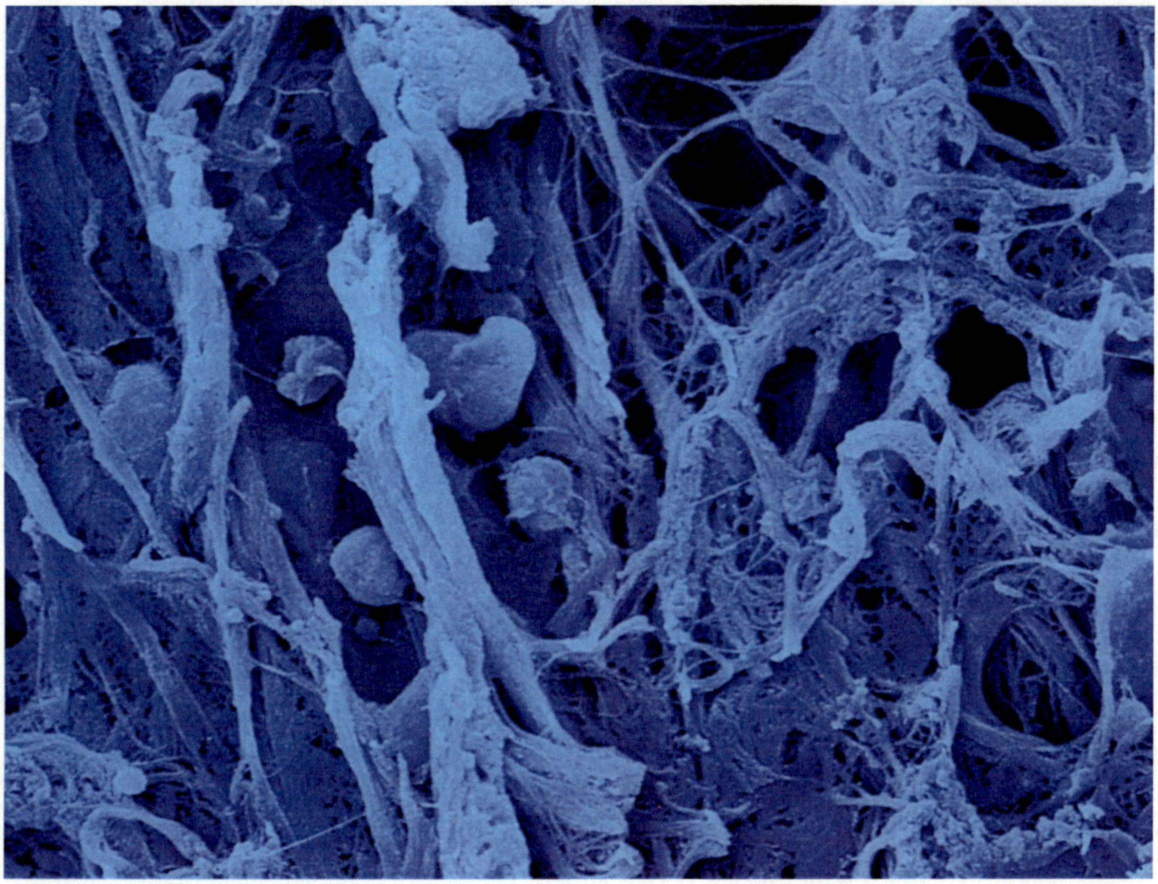

◁ Fig. 68
Advanced scarring in chronic pancreatitis. Inbetween tracts of collagen fibres scattered lymphocytes and variably large macrophages, some of which contain densely packed phagolysosomes. Narrow processes of fibroblasts. Variably broad, irregularly interlaced tracts of fibres in the surroundings.
Transmission electron micrograph
Magnification: 7500 ×

Fig. 69
Advanced scarring with extensive atrophy of the ductal system in chronic pancreatitis. Coarse fibre structure with irregularly intertwined tracts of collagen fibres. Scattered lymphocytes and macrophages located inbetween.
Scanning electron micrograph
Magnification: 2200 ×

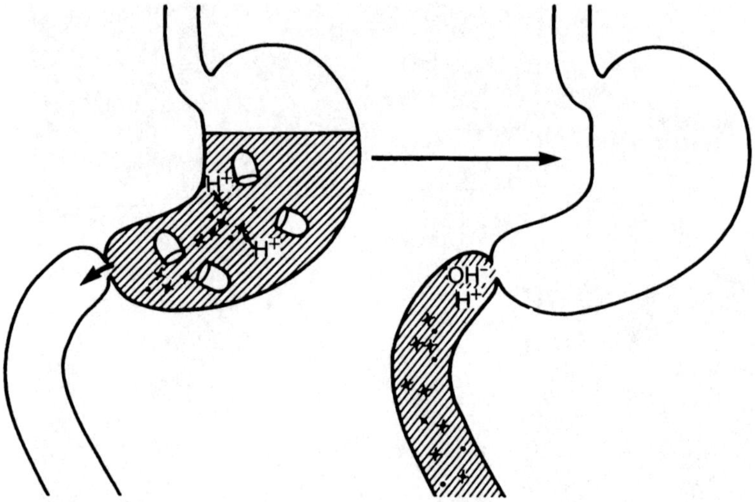

Inactivation of pancreatin (lipase!) by gastric acid

Insufficient lipase activity in the case of thorough mixing

a) Effect of pancreatin-preparations without acid-protective film: The lipase activity liberated in the stomach is partially inactivated by the acid and thus not sufficiently effective inspite of thorough mixing with the chymus.

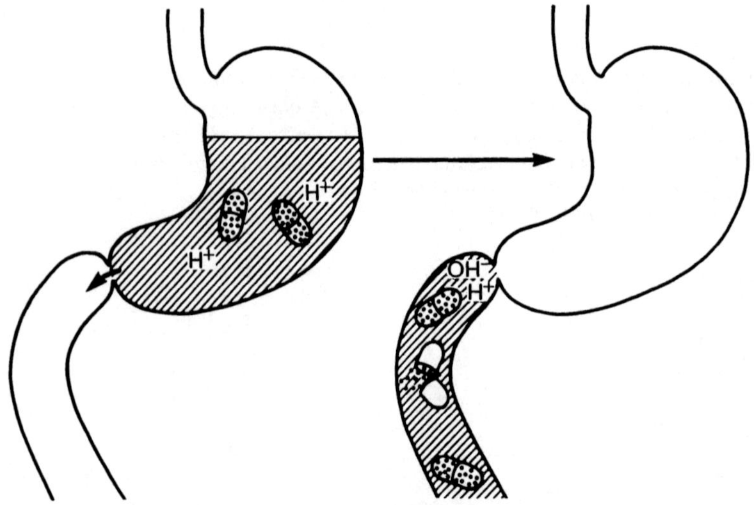

Pancreatin in acid-fast coat "enteric coat"

Intact lipase activity, but insufficient mixing

b) The effect of pancreatin-preparation in an acid-fast protective film. Inspite of preserved lipase activity in the gastric passage, cleavage of fat is still insufficient due to inadequate mixing of the chymus with the pancreatin.

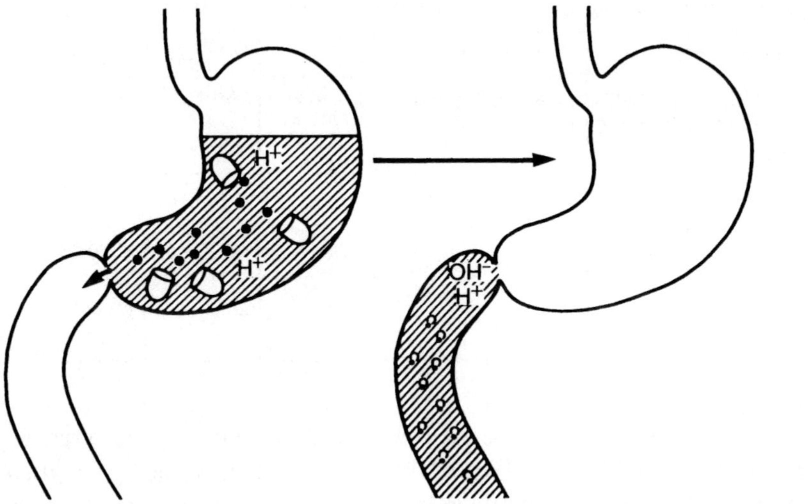

c) Mode of action of a microcapsulated pancreatin-preparation (e.g. Ureon®). The small acid-protected pancreatin granula are mixed with the chymus in the stomach and unfold their lipolytic activity in the alkaline environment of the upper small intestine.

Preparation selection and dose depend on the tolerance, the degree of steatorrhoea or as the case may be, the reduced chymotrypsin excretion in the stool.

The degree of success can be measured by clinical parameters such as reduction in stool weight, stool frequency and abating of flatulence and meteorism as well as in weight increase. If the desired success does not ensue, the diet and compliance of the patient should be looked into, the preparation possibly changed, or the dosage increased.

The different commercially available preparations differ not only in their lipase content, but also in their galenics and various additives. As a result of newer comparative studies modern pancreatin preparations, in which the lyophilized enzyme extract, derived mainly from swine pancreas, is packed in gastric acid resistant pellets are primarily recommended.

The small pellets are enclosed in a gelatine capsule easily dissolved in gastric secretions. Within a short period of time the swallowed capsule can dissolve in the stomach and the many little pellets are evenly distributed amongst the chymus (see Fig. a-c). The protective coat of the individual pellets prevent inactivation by gastric acid. The pellets, well mixed with the chymus and transported to the duodenum dissolve as of a pH value of 5.5 and release the enzyme activities. Additional blocking agents, e.g. with H2-receptor antagonists, as recommended earlier, are not necessary. In addition to the so-called late indication in established pancreoprive maldigestion in the course of chronic pancreatitis, a so-called early indication is subject of discussion. It has been advocated recently after demonstration in two controlled double-blind studies, that the pancreatic enzyme preparations ameliorate or even abort the pain in chronic pancreatitis, especially in the early phase of the disease, in which no exocrine pancreatic

Table 17 Effectivity of pancreatin preparations in the pain syndrome of chronic pancreatitis in two controlled studies

Author	Number	Type of Study	Preparation	Dose	Pain relief	Significance
Isaakson et al. 1983	n = 19	double blind against inactivated pancreatin	pancreatin granulate (Kreon®)	5× 7.5 ml	15/19	$p < 0.05$
Slaff et al. 1984	n = 20	placebo-double blind-crossover	pancreatin-granulate capsules	3×2+2x1	10/20	
	n = 12 of them without steatorrhoea				9/12	$p < 0.05$
	n = 8 with steatorrhoea				2/8	$p > 0.1$

insufficiency was apparent (Table 17). This pain-relieving effect is attributed to the negative feedback regulation of the trypsin content of the pancreatin. It is alleged that trypsin probably inhibits pancreatic secretion via nervous impulses upon contact with the mucosa of the upper small intestine, thus preventing postprandial pain. In preparation selection attention should thus be paid to the trypsin content apart from the lipase content and the galenics. As not all patients with chronic pancreatitis benefit from the early indication of pancreatic enzyme preparations for pain relief it is recommended that patients with chronic pancreatitis and painful episodes, even without evidence of exocrine pancreatic failure with steatorrhoea, ex juvantibus initially try pancreatic enzyme preparations in a dosage of 2–3 dragees or capsules each at mealtimes. If the desired pain-relief is not achieved the treatment can be stopped and not be indicated again until exocrine failure becomes manifest in later stages.

Diabetes mellitus

As pancreoprive diabetes mellitus is due to the exhaustion of insulin reserves oral antidiabetics are not effective as a rule. Dietetic management should take the necessary caloric intake of 240 to 300 easily degradable polysaccharides into account, regardless of simultaneous exocrine insufficiency. Daily blood glucose values of 160 to 200 mg % and sugar excretion in the urine exceeding 3 g per 24 h are indications for insulin supplementation. The blood glucose levels should not be maintained too low in view of the risk of hypoglycemia because of simultaneously reduced glucagon levels. Hypoglycemia is also aggravated by irregular food intake, e. g. owing to severe postprandial pain and by additional alcohol abuse and as the case may be discontinuation of pancreatic enzyme preparations.

Treatment of Pain (Table 18)

Table 18 Stepwise approach in the treatment of the pain syndrome in chronic pancreatitis

Step 1	▶ alcohol abstinence ▶ avoidance of animal-nutritive fats ▶ probatory enzymes
Step 2	▶ spasmoanalgesics/codeine phosphate paracetamol/(salicylates)
Step 3	▶ step 2 plus psychopharmaceutical drugs neuroleptics (Atosil®, Megaphen®) plus analeptics (Tofranil®, etc.)
Step 4	▶ opiate analogs (Temgesic®, Fortral®) plus combined neuroanaleptics (!)

Careful selection of the preparation and dosage are imperative for treatment of pain. In step I the general therapy must be checked for pain-relieving effects, such as alcohol elimination, frequent small meals, enzyme substitution (early indication!). For more severe pain episodes mainly peripherally effective analgesics such as paracetamol or salicylates, possibly in combination with codein phosphate are applied in stage II. The analgesic effect can be intensified by the simultaneous combined application of a neuroleptic such as triflupromazine or promethazine and an analeptic such as imipramine. Regular ingestion during painful episodes is important because analgesics can be saved in comparison to the prescription "when necessary". In step III the failure of the simple analgesics used in step II make substitution with opiate-analogs necessary. Due to the risk of toxomania care must be taken when assessing the situation, whether need really exists owing to the inflammatory episode or to pre-existing analgesic dependency. As a rule superimposing alcohol dependency aggravates the problem further. Upon failure of all these measures consideration should be given to elective surgery in therapy-resistent pain syndromes.

3.4.6.2 Surgical Therapy (Figs. 56, 70–73)

The advances in pancreatic diagnostics and the development of pancreatic surgery allow radical treatment of chronic pancreatitis in the same way it is performed regularly in case of pancreatic carcinoma. The indication for surgical treatment of chronic pancreatitis is determined by the occurrence of typical complications such as choledochal stenosis, stenosis of the duodenum, large cysts, ascites or pleural effusion (Kümmerle et al. 1979). It must be reckoned with these complications in about 20% of the cases of chronic pancreatitis. An indication for surgery is only applicable following a primarily conservative approach and consideration of all individual factors. Care must be taken to find the right moment for surgical intervention (Kümmerle et al. 1979). Particularly progressive cachexia must be taken into consideration. Early intervention can preserve the remaining endocrine and exocrine function. Systematic computerized tomographic observations have shown that spontaneous regression of pancreatic pseudocysts takes place in about 8% of the cases. In 30% secondary complications with bleeding or ruptures take place. Only close sequential sonographic evaluation of the dynamics of the cyst permit surgical measures in case of enlargement of the cyst. Biliary pancreatitis represents an absolute surgical indication, which, as a rule, can be brought to a standstill by correction of the bile ducts (Kümmerle et al. 1982). The preoperative assumption of the presence of pancreatic carcinoma also represents a surgical indication.

Especially the relative surgical indications, particularly the indication regarding the pain syndrome are controversial. The frequency reported for the occurrence of this complication in uncomplicated pancreatitis ranges between 4.3 (Ammann 1987) and 65% (Gebhard and Gall 1983). The pathogenesis of the pain is not sufficiently clear. Treatment can thus be given only on an empirical basis. It is assumed that the inflammatory alteration in the glandular tissue, the excess pressure in the pancreatic parenchyma lead to encasement of the sensory nerves or that the active perifocal inflammation surrounding the pseudocysts are the cause of the pain. Therapy-resistent pain can be assumed when morphologic alterations such as cysts or carcinomas are not evident and abuse of alcohol and narcotics can be excluded. It must be taken into consideration that in 20–50% new pancreatitis episodes can occur after pancreatic surgery.

Selection of the moment for surgery thus influences the post-operative result in respect to the success of the pain therapy. Long-term observations have shown that the best therapeutical results can be expected in late surgical intervention. 85% of the patients are free of pain after a median time period of 4 1/2 years (Beger 1985). Resection and autoamputation of the organ supplement each other in such a long course.

Essentially, the decision to perform surgery in chronic pancreatitis must be determined by the wish of the patient to cooperate and abstain from alcohol. Late mortalities as well as long-term complications depend mainly on postoperative continuation of alcohol abuse (Kozuschek et al. 1986). It is advocated that only the smallest possible and absolutely necessary surgical operation should be performed on uncooperative, injudicious alcoholics.

The surgical principles of treatment, which can be planned owing to improved diagnostic possiblities, depend on the local findings (Table 19).

Table 19 Indications for surgery (Kümmerle et al. 1979)

1. Absolute indications
– complications such as stenosis of the common bile duct, stenosis of the duodenum, large cysts
– ascites or
– pleural effusion
– chronic biliary pancreatitis
– suspicion of malignancy
2. Relative indications
– therapy-refractive pain syndrome
– therapy-resistent recurring episodes

Table 20 Methods of treatment

1	Resection procedures
1.1	Right lateral pancreatic resections
1.1.1	Partial right pancreatic resections, possibly with occlusion of the ducts
1.1.2	Total right pancreatic resections
1.1.3	Duodenum-preserving resection of the pancreatic head
1.2	Left lateral pancreatic resections
1.2.1	Partial left pancreatic resections (40–80%)
1.2.2	Subtotal left pancreatic resection (80–95%)
2	Drainage procedures
2.1	Internal drainage
2.1.1	Cysto-, jejuno-, duodeno- or gastrostomies
2.1.2	Drainage via the dilated pancreatic duct (Duval, Puestow)
2.2	External drainage (marsupialization)
3	Other Operations
3.1	Bile duct correction (cholecystectomy, revision of the common bile duct; cholecysto-, choledochojejunostomies, papillotomies)
3.2	Bypass operations
3.3	Nerve resection
3.4	Drainage of the pancreatic region
4	Conservative treatment
4.1	Avoidance of nutritive noxes
4.2	Medical treatment of endocrine and exocrine insufficiency
4.3	Analgesia

In a very dilated ductal system exceeding 8 mm in width and in large pancreatic cysts drainage methods are used. Puestow's pancreaticojejunostomy of a 10 to 12 cm portion of the small intestine with the 10 to 12 cm tail and body by means of a loop of defunctionalized small intestine with construction of an Roux en Y is performed. Intrapancreatic reflux should rarely occur.

When the pancreatic duct is dilated completely without stenosis Dural's approach presents itself. The essential condition for the appropriate drainage operation of the pancreatic ductal system is exact knowledge of the ductal morphology, which has either been revealed by preoperative ERCP or intraoperative visualization of the duct. Intraoperative sonography can be very helpful in finding the pancreatic duct (Avirdsson et al. 1985).

Purpose of internal drainage is decompression of the ductal system via a bypass or elimination of intraductal obstacles. Even though alterations in vicinity of the smaller tributary branches are not taken into account amelioration of pain occurs in 50 to 70% of the cases. The relatively poor late results of this method ensue from the persistence of the alterations within the small side branches. With progression of the disease further pancreatitic episodes occur. A carcinoma can also be overlooked when this method is applied.

The surgical procedure of choice for the pseudocysts appearing within the first 3 months subsequent to an acute episode are those utilizing drainage.

A cyst measuring more than 5 cm in diameter with a stable wall, capable of being anastomosed, should be operated because of the risk of rupture or infection or in case of pain ensuing from compression of adjacent organs. The method of choice is the cystojejunostomy as an anastomosis with a Roux en Y or a Braun-Entler jejunal anastomosis.

Depending on the local situation cystogastrostomies or cystoduodenostomies must be considered. The basic principle is to construct the broadest anastomosis possible at the deepest point taking the cyst contents into consideration. The pseudocysts consist of granulation tissue and a scarred zone enclosing a pool of blood, residues of haemorrhage, pancreatic enzymes and cell detritus (Edelmann et al. 1986). Even in the case of an endoanastomosis diversion of the complete pancreatic ductal system should be strived for as cysts can recur and the pancreatic pain continue. The presumption cannot be made that the pancreatic secretions can find an outlet into the jejunum via the

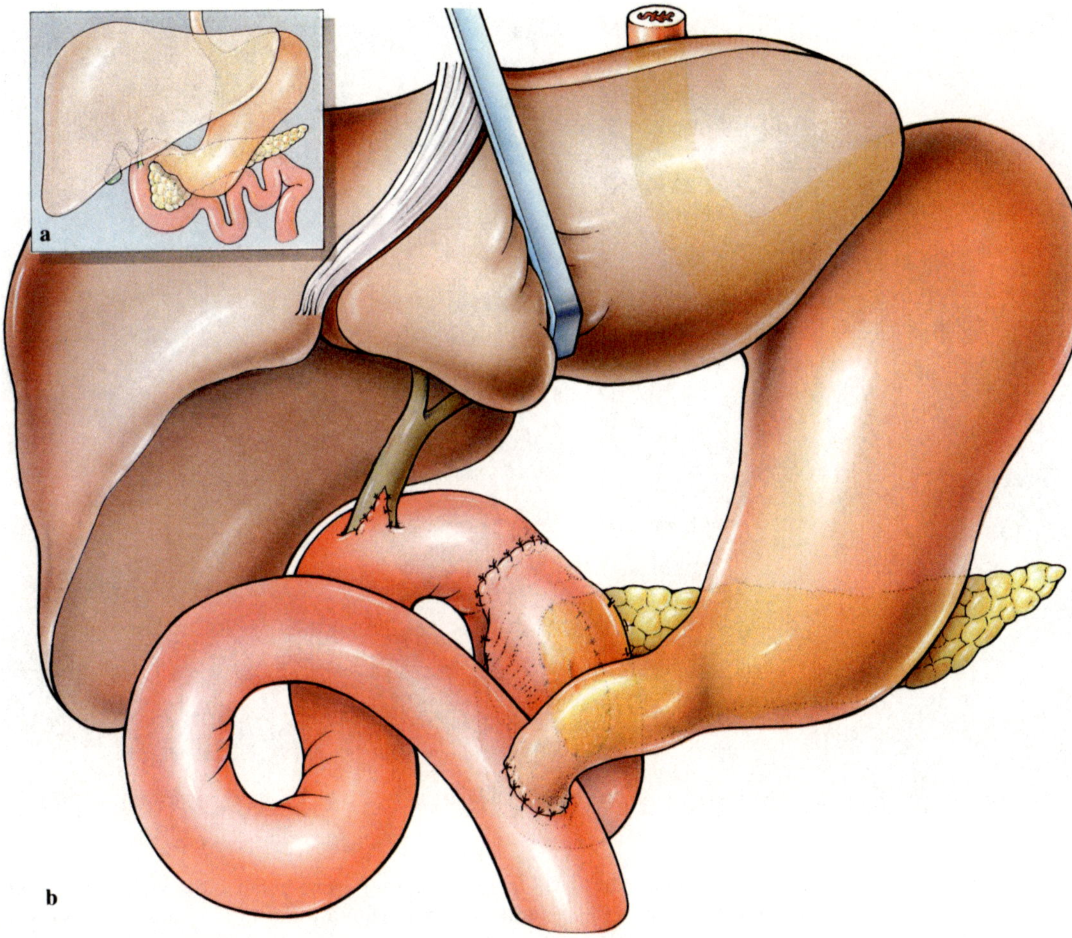

Fig. 70
Representation of the operation site in pylorus-preserving duodenopancreatectomy.
a) normal situs of the stomach, duodenum and pancreas
b) reconstruction after duodenopancreatectomy with retention of the pylorus and proximal duodenum. The terminolateral pancreatojejunostomy is enforced by a jejunoplication.

cyst as the connection usually obliterates after shrinkage of the cyst.

External drainage, either by introduction of a drain or stitching the cyst wall to the abdominal wound (marsupialisation), should be avoided because of long postoperative recovery periods in the case of large extrapancreatic pseudocysts. This procedure is mainly eligible in extremely large pseudocysts following an acute episode of pancreatitis. In this situation internal drainage is contraindicated because the wall of the cyst does not constitute a stable capsule, but only a fibrous, adhesive, flimsy wall formed by the neighboring organs (Hess 1969). Resection treatment must always be considered when pancreatic duct dilatations exceeding 8 mm diameter are missing. Ductal dilatation is evident in only 30% of the cases of pancreatitis (Krautzberger et al. 1985). Elimination of the inflammatory foci is a further consequent step in treatment, especially as these foci can be diagnosed better preoperatively with the new diagnostic procedures (Kümmerle et al. 1982).

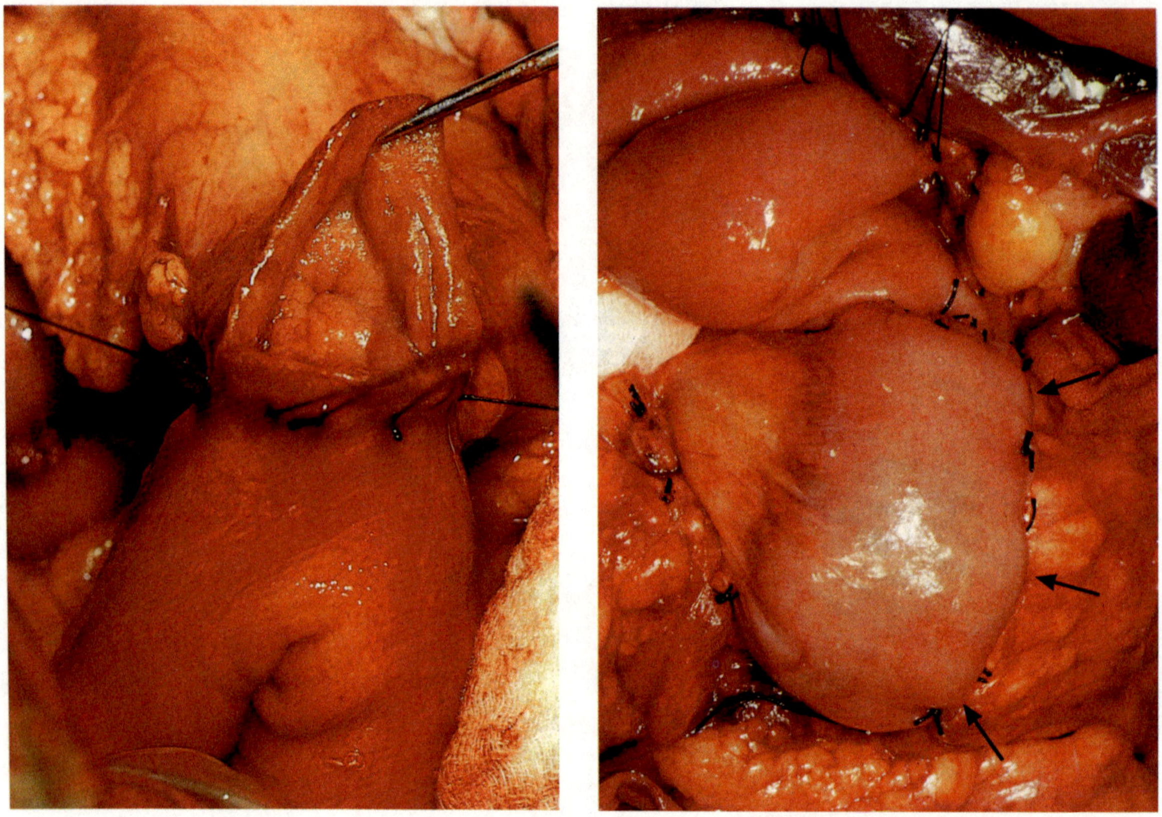

Fig. 71

a) Operation site following dissection of the duodenum in pylorus-preserving pancreatectomy. View into the proximal duodenum. Pylorus is closed. Perspective from caudal. The sero-serous sutures of the dorsal wall of the anastomosis (terminolateral) have been made and knotted.

b) Operation site following completion of the terminolateral pancreatojejunostomy with jejunoplication (arrows).

Of the operational procedures left lateral pancreatic resection, which preserves the duodenum must be distinguished from right lateral pancreatoduodenal resection, which additionally intervenes in the physiological transportation pathway of nutrients. Depending on the extent of pancreatic resection partial or total, or in some cases subtotal measures are distinguished from one another. Partial left lateral pancreatic resections and subtotal left lateral pancreatic resections, which technically extend across the vascular ligament to the median, are justified in segmental pancreatitis in the pancreatic tail and on occasion in this connection thrombosis of the splenic vein with segmental or portal hypertension (Krautzberger et al. 1985).

Right lateral pancreatic resection, Whipple's classic partial duodenopancreatectomy (1935) is performed in the treatment of severe pancreatitis with development of an inflammatory tumor of the pancreatic head. Every duodenopancreatectomy consists of three operational phases:

1. Exploration
2. Mobilization and Resection
3. Reconstruction of gastrointestinal and biliodigestive continuity.

During exploration it must be illuminated whether the tumorous pancreatitis of the pancreatic head is operable. An inflammatory or even tumorous encasement of the superior mesentery vein or enclo-

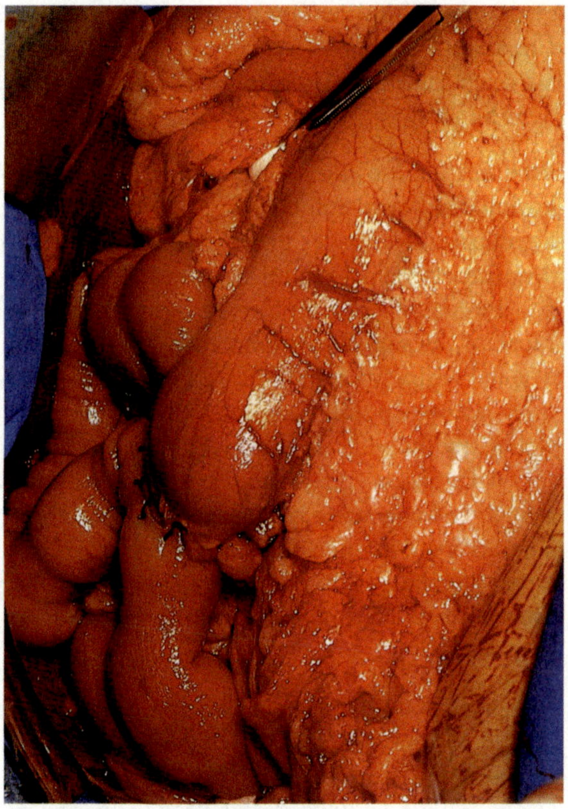

Fig. 72
Duodenopancreatic head resection with preservation of the stomach and pylorus. Operation site after completion of all anastomoses.

sure of the portal vein exclude radical pancreatic head resection.

In Whipple's procedure pancreatic head resection, resection of the distal 2/3 of the stomach, the duodenum, the main bile duct including the cystic duct and the gallbladder as well as the first 10 to 15 cm of the proximal jejunum are mandatory for anatomical and physiological reasons. Reconstruction of the continuity begins after the resection of the pancreatic head with the anastomosis between the pancreatic rest and the jejunum. This anastomosis is the cause of possible complications such as suture disruption as well as the risk of inflammation of the remaining pancreas.

The risk of disruption of the pancreatic anastomosis can be prevented by wide plication of the jejunum around the terminolateral pancreatojejunal anastomosis (Siedeck et al. 1985, Kozuschek 1985, 1986). Depending on the consistency of the pancreatic parenchyma and the morphology of the duct in the remaining pancreas various techniques for constructing anastomoses have been applied. Right lateral pancreatic resection can be combined with construction of a pancreatojejunal anastomosis (Horn 1987). Intraoperative duct occlusion with an organic, intraductal hardening prolamin solution (Ethibloc) is advocated as a further measure to stabilize the pancreatic anastomosis and prevent further complaints or recurrence (Gebhardt 1984).

The extension of Whipple's operation to complete removal of the organ – total duodenopancreatectomy – involves complete loss of endocrine and exocrine pancreatic function. Operational risk, postoperative complications and late operative morbidity have a positive correlation to the large trauma to the organ (Raupach 1986).

Whipple's partial duodenopancreatectomy is associated with a high postoperative mortality rate and bad digestive function. The high mortality could be attributed to the lacking experience of the surgeons and the dangerous pancreatic anastomosis in the past. Both factors have been corrected since.

In order to improve the postoperative digestive function following duodenopancreatectomy Traverso and Longmire (1978, 1980) recommended preservation of the stomach, pylorus and proximal duodenum. In the mean time more than 252 cases have been reported, in which the operation procedure has been applied (Braasch et al. 1986). Judging by our own experience with 23 patients pylorus-preservation has proven to be an advantageous operational procedure (Kozuschek 1985, Edelmann and Kozuschek 1986).

In this surgical technique the procedure is similar to that of standard pancreatectomy. The duodenum is dissected 2 to 4 cm distal to the pylorus. As the right gastroepiploic artery, the inferior pancreatoduodenal artery and the right gastric artery must be ligated in pancreatic head resection, the arterial supply of the duodenal stump succeeds via the left gastric artery along the small curvature of the stomach and the pylorus. It is thus imperative to preserve this vasculature, as suture disruption arises otherwise. Latarjet's nerve plexus, which innervates the antrum and pylorus must be preserved. The duodenum is implanted end-to-side in the jejunum limb, which has been pulled up to the biliary anastomosis and the pancreatic anastomosis. The advantages of pylorus preservation in duodenopancreatectomy are convincing and have the following reasons:

1. The operation is limited to the right upper abdomen and thus the
2. operational trauma is less and the duration of the operation is shorter and
3. the anatomy warranting digestion and nutrition are improved postoperatively.

The postoperative gastroenteral passage shows no conspicuous findings. Gastric atony is observed very rarely (Kozuschek 1985). The pyloric function is unimpaired judging by radiological and endoscopical findings. Follow-ups established that no problems arise in regard to maldigestion and malabsorption (Edelmann and Kozuschek 1986). By preserving the antropyloric and bulbar units some mechanisms aiding digestion are partially, some are completely maintained. The para- and endocrine functional unit is not completely destroyed. Entero-gastrin-secretin, cholecysto- and pancreatokinin are still released from the remaining parts of the duodenum (Braasch et al. 1986). The neuroendocrine functional unit is present to a large extent. The enzyme secretory regulation can adapt to the new situation and replenish itself. The remaining pancreas can take over its function without exhibiting essential signs of insufficiency, as long as not more than 90% was resected.

Following pylorus-preserving procedures the ulcer rate is extremely low in an overview of the literature. It equals 2 to 3% (Kozuschek 1985, Itani et al. 1986). The ulcers occurred mainly in patients who underwent total pancreatectomy. Gebhard et al. (1982) and Gall (1979), who added occlusion of the pancreatic duct to the pylorus-preserving pancreatectomy, thus deliberately forfeiting exocrine pancreatic function characterized by secretion of bufferent substances, observed an ulcer frequency of 39%.

Whether the low ulcer rate can be confirmed following long-term follow-up remains to be seen. Significant differences in the postoperative complication rate in pylorus-preservation and standard pancreatectomy can not be registered to date because of the small case numbers as yet. The most frequent cause of complications are disruption of the anastomosis both in vicinity of the pancreas as well as the bile ducts. Jejunoplication in conjunction with the pancreatic anastomosis reduced the rate of clinically manifest suture disruption almost completely. The mortality rates can not be compared objectively to date. Until now mortality rates of the pylorus-preserving operation have not been compared.

The basis of every therapy of chronic pancreatitis are the conservative measures, which aside from the elimination of pain and the prevention of relapses aim for a compensation of the exocrine and endocrine pancreatic insufficiency. The indication for surgical intervention lies primarily in the complications of the disease, which are responsible for a great deal of the deaths ensuing from this form of the disease. To what extent operational procedures will influence the course of this disease in the future depend on the selected procedure itself, avoidance of the most frequent risk factor, alcohol abuse, and the stage of the disease.

In surgical therapy of chronic pancreatitis the resecting procedures have increasingly banished the drainage methods during the past few years because of the better results in amelioration of pain. It must be taken into consideration that a general preference of one of both principles of treatment – drainage or resection – is not justified because in each individual case the most adequate operational technique must be selected for each individual course.

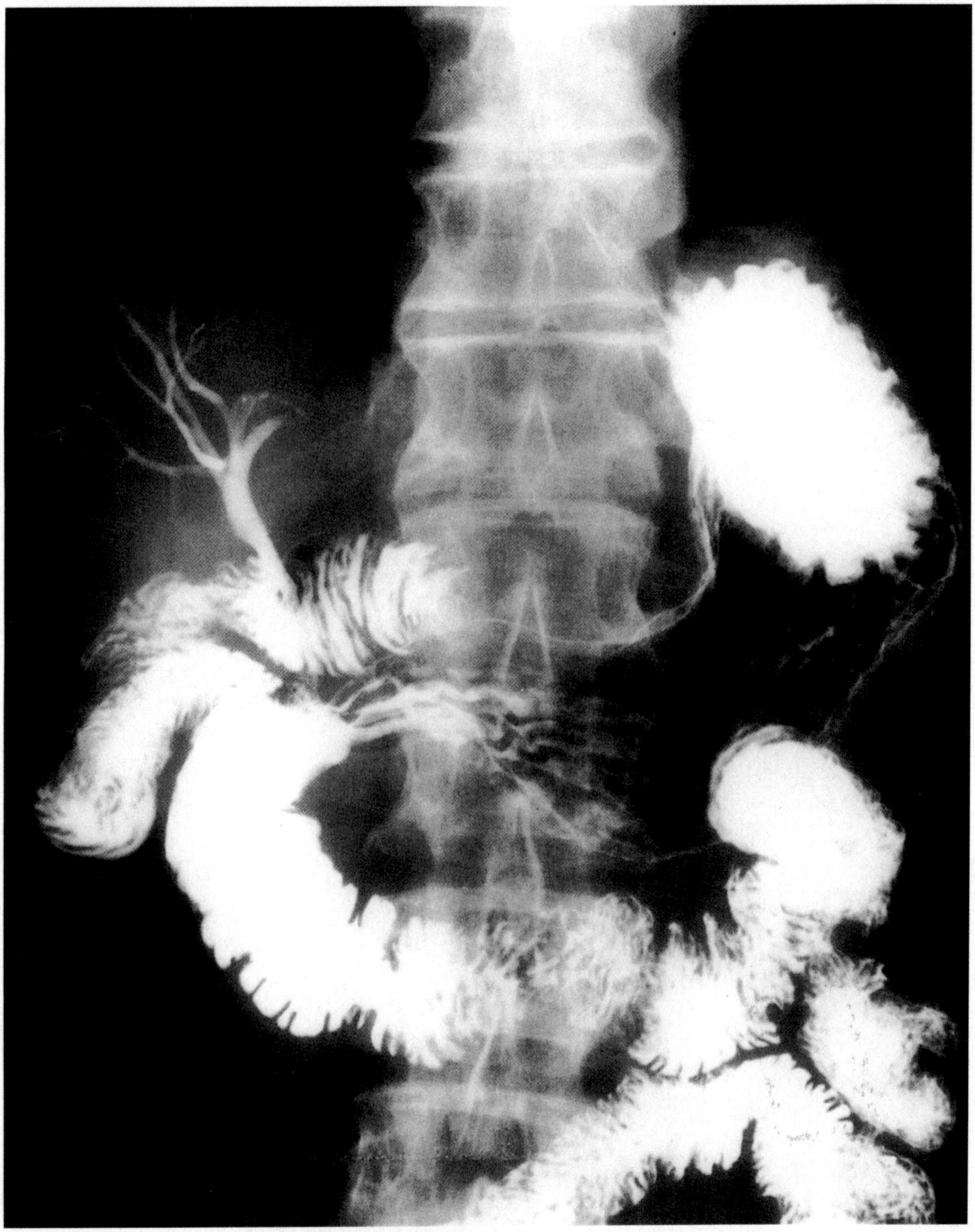

Fig. 73
Control x-ray examination 14 days after duodenopancreatic head resection with pylorus-preservation. Depiction of the anastomoses to the residual pancreas, bile duct and proximal duodenum. Strong peristalsis of the gastric antrum and unimpaired pyloric function.

4 References

Acosta, J.M., Ledesma, C.L. (1974) Gallstone Migration as a cause of acute Pancreatitis. New Engl. J. Med. 290, 484

Ammann, R. (1987) Chronische Pankreatitis: Definition, Schweregrad und therapeutische Konsequenzen. Chirurg 58, 1

Arendt, R., Moldenhauer, W., Hauzeur, F., Kröger, W. (1979) Der Beitrag der ERCP zur Diagnostik der chronischen Pankreatitis. Z. ges. Inn. Med. 34, 286

Avirdsson, S., Grendl, S., Ohlsson, K., Wehlin, L. (1985) Experience of surgical treatment for chronic pancreatitis during a 10-year period. Acta Chir. Scand. 151, 267

Balser, W. (1882) Über Fettnekrose, eine zuweilen tödliche Krankheit des Menschen. Arch. path. Anat. 90, 520

Becker, V. (1984) Chronische Pankreatitis – Klinische Morphologie. Thieme, Stuttgart, New York

Beger, H.G. (1985) Neue Aspekte in der Pankreaschirurgie. Klinikarzt 14, 228

Bernard, C. (1856) Lecons de physiologic experimentale appliquée a la medictue. Baillére, Paris

Bohnsack, R., Kozuschek, W., Bittscheidt, H., Singbartl. G. (1983) Intensivmedizinische und chirurgische Maßnahmen bei der Behandlung der akuten Pankreatitis. Intensivmedizin 20, 67

Borchard, F. (1987) Gallenwege und Pankreas. Verh. Dtsch. Ges. Path. 71, 53

Braasch, J.W., Gongliang, J., Rossi, R.L. (1984) Pancreatoduodenectomy with preservation of the pylorus. World J. Surg. 8, 900

Braasch, J.W., Deziel, D.J., Rossi, R.L., Watkins, E., Winter, P.F. (1986) Pyloric and Gastric Preserving Pancreatic Resection. Experience with 87 Patients. Ann. Surg. 204, 411

Büchler, M., Krautzberger, W., Block, S., Beger, H.G. (1985) Neue Aspekte in der Chirurgie der akuten Pankreatitis. Der Klinikarzt 14, 455–466

Bünte, H. (1971) Pankreatitis nach Magenresektion. Langenbecks Arch. Chir. 329, 1054

Chiari, H. (1896) Über Selbstverdauung des menschlichen Pankreas. Z. Heilk. (Prag) 17, 69

Classen, W. (1984) Erkrankungen des Pankreas. In: W. Siegenthaler, W. Haufmann, H. Hornhostel, H.D. Wallner (Hrsg.): Lehrbuch der inneren Medizin Thieme, Stuttgart, New York

Colmant, H.J., Noltenius, H. (1977) Pankreatische Enzephalopathie. Med. Klin. 72, 2146

Creutzfeld, W. (1977) Erkrankungen der Bauchspeicheldrüse. In: Gross, R. (Hrsg.), Schölmerich, P. (Hrsg.): Lehrbuch der inneren Medizin. Schattauer-Verlag, Stuttgart, New York

Creutzfeld, W. (1987) Pathophysiologie des endokrinen Pankreas. Verh. Dtsch. Ges. Path. 71, 16

Dammann, H.G., Grabbe, E. (1981) Klinische, laborchemische und computertomographische Charakterisierung des vital bedrohten Patienten bei der akuten Pankreatitis. Leber, Magen, Darm 11, 174

Dammann, H.G., Döpner, M. (1981) Die Beurteilung der Frühdiagnose der akuten Pankreatitis. Zentralblatt der Chirurgie, 106, 154

Dammann, H.G., Grabbe, E., Brockmann, W.P., Klöppel, G. (1982) Diagnostik bei chronischer Pankreatitis – Sicherer Nachweis erst im fortgeschrittenen Stadium. Klinikarzt 11, 250

Dürr, G.H.K. (1979) Acute pancreatitis. In: Howat, H.T., Sarles, H. (Hrsg.): The Exocrine Pancreas. Saunders, Philadelphia, 352–401

Edelmann, M., Pelzer, Ch., Kozuschek, W. (1985) Die temporäre tangentiale Ileostomie und die programmierte Laparotomie – zwei Möglichkeiten eines sinnvollen Konzeptes in der chirurgischen Behandlung der schweren Peritonitis. Langenbecks Arch. (Kongreßbericht), 630

Edelmann, M., Kozuschek, W., Kozianka, J. (1986) Pankreaspseudozysten – Diagnostik, Chirurgische Therapie. In: Kozuschek, W. (Hrsg.) Chirurgische Klinik 1975–1985. Bundesknappschaft Bochum, 124

Edelmann, M., Kozuschek, W. (1986) Preservation of the Pylorus in Pancreatiduodenectomy. 9th World Congress Collegium Internationale Digestivae, Jerusalem 31.08.–05.09.1986. Dig. Surg. 3, 88 (Abstract)

Farthmann, E.H., Männl, H.F.K. (1980) Postoperative Pankreatitis – Übersicht. In: Häring, R. (Hrsg.): Die akute und chronische Pankreatitis. TM-Verlag, Bad Oeynhausen, 129

Ferner, H. (1979) Die Bauchspeicheldrüse. In: H. Ferner, J. Staubesand: Benninghoff/Goertler; Lehrbuch der Anatomie des Menschen. Bd. 2, 12. Aufl. Eingeweide und Kreislauf. Urban und Schwarzenberg, München

Fitz, R.H. (1889) Acute Pancratitis: A Consideration of Pancreatic Hemorrhage, Hemorrhagic, Suppurative and Gangrenous Pancreatitis and of Disseminated Fat. Necrosis. Boston Med. Surg. J. 120, 181

Forell, M.M. (1979) Diagnostisches Vorgehen bei der chronischen Pankreatitis unter Berücksichtigung der Aussagekraft der einzelnen Methoden. Internist 20, 360

Friedrich, N. (1878) Disease of the Pancreas. In: Ziemsen,

H. (Hrsg.): Cyclopedia of the Practice of Medicine. Wm. Wood & Co., New York, 8, 599

Fritsch, A. (1980) Akute Pankreatitis-Indikationen, Verfahrenswahl und Ergebnisse der operativen Behandlung. Chirurg 51 (6), 376

Gall, F.P. Gebhardt, C. (1979) Ein neues Konzept in der Chirurgie der chronischen Pankreatitis. Dtsch. Med. Wochenschr. 104, 1003

Gebhardt, Ch., Gall, F.P., Rösch, W., Schackert, H.K. (1982) Anastomosenulkus nach Whipple-Operation mit Magenerhaltung. Zbl. Chir. 107, 952

Gebhardt, Ch. (1984) Chirurgische Therapie der chronischen Pankreatitis. In: Gebhardt, Ch. (Hrsg.): Chirurgie des exokrinen Pankreas. Georg Thieme, Stuttgart New York, 139

Gmelin, E., Weiss, H.-D., Fuchs, H.-D., Reiser M. (1981) Vergleich der diagnostischen Treffsicherheit von Ultraschall. Computertomografie und ERCP bei der chronischen Pankreatitis und beim Pankreaskarzinom.

Goebell, H. (1980) Ätiologie und Pathogenese der akuten und chronischen Pankreatitis. In: Chirurgie der akuten und chronischen Pankreatitis. Hrsg. Häring, R., TM-Verlag, Bad Oeynhausen, 11

Goebell, H., Dürr, G.H.K. (1981) Akute Pankreatitis – Pro und Contra der modernen Therapie. Internist 22, 684–693

Hentschel, A. (1978) Pankreas. In: Lehrbuch der Chirurgie. Koslowski, L. (Hrsg.), Irmer, W. (Hrsg.), Buhse, K.A. (Hrsg.) Schattauer Verlag, Stuttgart, New York

Hess, W. (1969) Die chronische Pankreatitis, H. Huber Bern – Stuttgart

Hoefler, H. (1979) Pankreasnekrose: Todesursache, Überlebenszeit und Wahl des Operationszeitpunktes. DMW 104, 315

Hoffmann, R., Berthold, S. (1979) Akute hämorrhagische Pankreatitis. Helv. Chir. Acta 46, 593

Hoffmeister, A.W., Trede, M. (1982) Chronisch rezidivierende Pankreatitis – Chirurgische Therapie individuell planen. Klinikarzt 11, 271

Hollender, L.F. (1979) Resection of the pancreas for acute hemorrhagic et necrotizing pancreatitis. World J. Surg., 3, 637

Hollender, L.F., Lehnert, P., Wanke, M. (1983) Akute Pankreatitis. Urban & Schwarzenberg. München, Wien, Baltimore

Horn, J. (1983) Das Ileostoma als Teil des chirurgischen Therapiekonzeptes bei der akuten Pankreatitis. Chirurg 54, 320

Horn, J., Hohenberger, P. (1987) Chronische Pankreatitis – Drainage und Resektionsverfahren. Standortbestimmung. Chirurg 58, 14

Hotz, J., Schwemmle, K. (1984) Chronische Pankreatitis – Konsequenzen und praktisches Vorgehen. In: Goebell, H., Hotz, K., Farthmann, E.H. (Hrsg.): Der chronisch Kranke in der Gastroenterologie. Springer, Berlin, 235–246

Howard, J.M., Jordan, G.L. (1956) Relapsing pancreatitis secondary to choledocholithiasis. A.M.A. Arch. Surg. 73, 960

Huck, L., Knop. P., Hausamen. T.U. (1981) Sonografische Pankreasdiagnose bei unklaren Oberbauchbeschwerden. DMW 106, 71

Isaksson, G., Ihse, I. (1983) Pain reduction by an oral pancreatic enzyme preparation in chronic pancreatitis. Dig. Dis. Sci. 28, 97

Itani, K.M.F., Coleman, R.E., Akwari, O.E., Meyers, W.C. (1986) Pylorus – preserving Pancreatoduodenectomy. A clinical and physiologicappriabal. Ann. Surg. 204, 655

Kern, E. (1980) Pankreaschirurgie. In: Zenker, Deucher, Schink (Hrsg.): Chirurgie der Gegenwart. Urban Schwarzenberg, München, Wien, Baltimore, Bd. 7, 51

Kern, H.F. (1987) Kompartimentierung und Proteintransport in der Azinuszelle des Pankreas als pathophysiologisches Konzept. Verh. Dtsch. Ges. Path. 71, 24

Klose, J., Neher, M., Kümmerle, F. (1983) Operative Behandlung bei der akuten Pankreatitis. DMW 108, 490

Klöppel, G. (1984) Islet histopathology in diabetes mellitus. In: G. Klöppel, Ph. u. Heitz (Eds.) Pancreatic pathology. Churchill Livingstone London

Körte, W. (1894) Zur chirurgischen Behandlung der Pankreas-Eiterung und Pankreas-Nekrose. Arch. klin. Chir. 48, 720

Kozuschek, W. (1979) Geschwülste des Pankreas. In: Kampf dem Krebs. Nr. 19. Arbeitsgemeinschaft für Krebsbekämpfung der gesetzlichen Krankenkassen und Rentenversicherung NRW (Hrsg.), Bochum, 40

Kozuschek, W. (1985) Pancreaticoduodenectomy with Pylorus Preservation, 5th African Federation Congress, Int. Coll. Surg. 25.11.–28.11.85 Kairo, 73 (Abstract)

Kozuschek, W. (1986) Pankreas. In: Kozuschek, W. (Hrsg.) Chirurgische Klinik 1975–1985. Bundesknappschaft Bochum, 56

Kozuschek, W., Bohnsack, R., Edelmann, M., Raupach, W. (1986) Langzeitergebnisse nach operativer Behandlung der chronischen Pankreatitis. In: Kozuschek, W. (Hrsg.): Chirurgische Klinik 1975–1985, Bundesknappschaft Bochum, 134

Krautzberger, W., Büchler, M., Berger, H.-G. (1985) Neue Aspekte in der Chirurgie der chronischen Pankreatitis. Klinikarzt 14, 378

Kümmerle, F., Mannegold, G., Rückert, K. (1979) Chirurgie des Pankreas – Chronische Pankreatitis, Pankreaskarzinom, endokrine Pankreastumoren. Internist 20, 399

Kümmerle, F., Frick, S., Günther, R. (1982) Tendenzen in der Chirurgie der chronischen Pankreatitis. DMW 107, 531

Lackner, K., Frommhold, H., Grauthoff, H., Mödder, U., Heuser, L., Braun, G., Buurman, R., Scherer, K. (1980) Wertigkeit der Computertomografie und der Sonografie innerhalb der Pankreasdiagnostik. Fortschr. Röntgenstr. 132, 509

Langmann, J. (1979) Pankreas. In: Langmann, J. (Hrsg.) Medizinische Embryologie: Thieme Stuttgart

Lankisch, P. G., Lopez, E., Winckler, K., Schuster, R. (1976) Kolonstenosen nach Pankreatitis. Schweiz. med. Wschr. 106, 1243

Lankisch, P. G., Ehrhardt-Schmelzer, S. (1984) Die Chymotrypsinbestimmung im Stuhl: Ein indirekter Pankreasfunktionstest. DMW 109, 1527

Lindner, H. (1964) Akute Pankreatitis (Pankreasnekrose) infolge Glucocorticoidtherapie. DMW 89, 833

Mallet-Guy, P., Giura, F. (1957) Reflux Wirsungien et pancreatites, Analyse d' une deuxieme serie de 400 cas de reflux cholangiographique dans canal de Wirsung. Lyon. Chir. 53, 481

Malfertheiner, P., Feurle, G. E., Büchler, M., Kemmer, T., Ditschuneit, H. (1984) Chronische Pankreatitis – Diagnostische Bedeutung des pankreatischen Polypeptids. MMW 126, 1183

Marks, I. N., Bank, S., Barbezat, G. O. (1976) Alkoholpankreatitis – Ätiologie, klinische Formen, Komplikationen. Leber Magen Darm 6, 257

Mellmann, J., Fuchs, R., Helenius, A. (1986) Acidification of the endocytic and exocytic pathways. Ann. Rev Biochem. 55, 663

Neher, M., Kümmerle, F., Klose, K. J. (1982) Der Einfluß von Sonographie und Computertomographie auf die operative Behandlung der akuten Pankreatitis. Langenbecks Arch. klin. Chir. 356, 141

Neher, M., Kümmerle, F., Klose, K. J. (1977) Verzögerte Operationen bei akuter Pankreatitis. Chir. 48, 439

Neher, M., Manegold, G., Rückert, K., Kümmerle, F. (1980) Möglichkeiten und Grenzen der Pankreaschirurgie. DMW 75, 613

Otte, M. (1979) Pankreasfunktionsdiagnostik. Internist 20, 331

Palade, G. E. (1975) Intracellular aspects of the process secretion. Sience 189, 347

Phat, V. N., Guerrieni, M. F., Alexandre, J. H., Camilleri, J. P. (1984) Early histological changes in acute necrotizing hemorrhagic pancreatis. Path. Res. Pract. 178, 273

Radke, R., Radke, M., Radke, C. (1985) Licht- und elektronenmikroskopische Untersuchungen zur Innervation des exokrinen Pankreas. Z. mikr.-anat. Forsch. 99, 735

Ranson, J. H. (1978) Prognostic signs and nonoperative peritoneal lavage in acute pancreatitis. Ann. surg. 187, 565

Rao, K. N., Zuretti, M. F., Baccino, F. M., Lombardi, B. (1980) Acute hemorrhagic pancreatic necrosis in mice. Am. J. Pathol. 89, 45

Raupach, W. (1986) Aktive Therapie in der Behandlung der chronischen Pankreatitis. Ergebnisse und Verlauf, Krankengut der Chirurgischen Universitätsklinik Bochum, Knappschaftskrankenhaus der Jahre 1976–1983. Bochum, Dissertation

Remmele, W. (1984) Exokrines Pankreas. In: W. Remmele (Hrsg.) Pathologie. Springer, Berlin, Heidelberg, New York, Tokyo

Rinderknecht, H. (1986) Pancreatic secretory enzymes. In: V. L. W. Go et al. (Eds): The exocrine pancreas. Biology, Pathobiology, and Disease. Raven Press, New York

Roggenwallner, B. (1985) Die chirurgische Behandlung der hämorrhagisch-nekrotisierenden Pankreatitis – Ergebnisse der chirurgischen Behandlung mit Berücksichtigung des Spätstatus bei 44 im Knappschafts-Krankenhaus Bochum-Langendreer in der Zeit von 1977 bis 1984 operierten Patienten, Bochum, Dissertation

Rösch, W., Haschke, H., Phillip, J. (1981) Lebenserwartung bei chronischer Pankreatitis. Lebenversicherungsmedizin 33, 87

Rösch, W. (1983) Operative Behandlung der chronischen Pankreatitis. Z. Gastroenterologie 21, 181

Rothmann, J. E., (1987) Proteinsorting by selective retention in the endoplasmatic reticulum and golgi stack. Cell 50, 521

Sarles, H. (1965) Symposium Marseille 25./26. April 1963. Karger, Basel New York

Sarles, J.-C., Sarles, H. (1976) Konservative und chirurgische Therapie der chronischen Pankreatitis. Leber Magen Darm 6, 294

Sarles, H., Cros, R. C., Bidard, J. M. (1979) A Multicenter Inquiry into the Etiology of Pancreatic Diseases. Digestion (Basel) 19, 1110

Schalimov, A. A., Schalimov, S. A., Zemskov, W. S., Podprjatov, E. E. (1980) Zur Behandlungstaktik der akuten Pankreatitis. Zentralblatt f. Chir. 105, 842

Schiebler, T. H. (1987) Zur Biologie der Bauchspeicheldrüse. Verh. Dtsch. Ges. Path. 71, 1

Schirmer, S. (1893) Beitrag zur Geschichte des Pankreas. Basel, Dissertation

Schmidt, R. F., Thews, G. (1980) Physiologie des Menschen. Springer, Berlin, Heidelberg, New York

Schmitz-Moormann, P. (1987) Chronische Pankreatitis. Morphologie und Pathogenese. Verh. Dtsch. Ges. Path. 71, 161

Schuster, H. P., Neher, M., Schönborn, H., Kümmerle, F. (1980) Akutes Nieren- und Lungenversagen bei diffuser Peritonitis und hämorrhagisch-nekrotisierender Pankreatitis. DMW 105, 82

Siedek, M., Birtel, F., Mitrenga, I. (1985) Pankreasanastomose und Pankreatojejunoplicatio nach Rechtsresektion. Langenbecks Arch. (Kongreßbericht) 610

Siegenthaler, W. (1976) Klinische Pathophysiologie. Thieme-Verlag, Stuttgart, 833

Singer, M.V., Gyr, K., Sarles, H. (1985) Revidierte Marseille-Klassifikation der Pankreatitis. Deutsches Ärzteblatt 82, 116

Slaff, J., Jacobson, D., Tillman, C.R., Curington, C., Toskes, P. (1984) Proteasespecific suppression of pancreatic exocrine secretion. Gastroenterology 87, 44–52

Stolte, M. (1987) Chronische Pankreatitis. Verh. Dtsch. Ges. Path. 71, 175

Stömmer, P. (1987) Pankreaserkrankungen und andere Organe. Verh. Dtsch. Ges. Path. 71, 68

Traverso, L.W., Longmire, W.P. (1978) Preservation of the pylorus in pancreaticoduodenectomy. Surg. Gynecol. Obstet 146, 959

Traverso, L.W., Longmire, W.P. (1980) Preservation of the pylorus in pancreaticoduodenectomy: A follow – up evaluation. Ann. Surg. 192, 306

Volkholz, H.M., Stolte (1984) Pathologie der Pseudozysten. In: Chirurgie des exokrinen Pankreas. Hrsg. Gehbardt, Ch., Georg Thieme Stuttgart, 69

Whipple, A.O., Parsons, W.B., Mullins, C.R. (1935) Treatment of carcinoma of the ampulla of Vater. Ann. Surg. 144, 612